THE GREAT PHYSICIAN'S

Rx *for*

WEIGHT LOSS

JORDAN RUBIN

with Joseph Brasco, M.D.

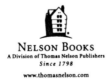

NELSON BOOKS
A Division of Thomas Nelson Publishers
Since 1798

www.thomasnelson.com

Copyright © 2006 by Jordan S. Rubin

All rights reserved. No portion of this book may be reproduced, stored in a retrieval system, or transmitted in any form or by any means—electronic, mechanical, photocopy, recording, scanning, or other—except for brief quotations in critical reviews or articles, without the prior written permission of the publisher.

Published in Nashville, Tennessee, by Thomas Nelson, Inc.

Nelson Books titles may be purchased in bulk for educational, business, fund-raising, or sales promotional use. For information, please e-mail SpecialMarkets@ThomasNelson.com.

Scripture quotations are from the New King James Version®. Copyright © 1979, 1980, 1982 by Thomas Nelson, Inc. Used by permission. All rights reserved.

Library of Congress Cataloging-in-Publication Data

Rubin, Jordan.
    The Great Physician's Rx for weight loss / by Jordan Rubin with Joseph Brasco.
      p. cm.
    Includes bibliographical references (p.   ).
      ISBN: 0785297499

    1. Weight loss. 2. Weight loss—Religious aspects—Christianity. I. Brasco, Joseph. II. Title.
RM222.2.R814 2006
613.2'5—dc22   2005036824

Printed in the United States of America

07 08 09 10 QW 10 9

To all the people who look in the mirror and know they are not experiencing all of the health that God intended for them. May this book inspire you to present your bodies as living sacrifices. God will do the rest.

CONTENTS

INTRODUCTION

A Mighty Turnaround

Doris Bailey, fifty-six years old, remembers the incident like it happened yesterday.

She was just fifteen, a young woman trying to find her place in a big world, but acutely aware of rejection and not having any friends. She was diminutive in stature—just five feet, two inches tall—but carrying too much weight at 185 pounds. At school, Doris preferred to remain in the background, where she wouldn't be noticed—or rejected. "I was a loner, someone who stayed by myself," she recalls.

One evening she was home when her older brother, Sonny, a senior in high school, invited some of his buddies to hang out. The boys were cutting up and joking around when one of them caught Doris's eye.

"Hey, Doris, want an apple?" he asked. He reached for a shiny Red Delicious stacked in a bowl of fruit on the dining room table.

"Sure," Doris responded, not giving the question a second thought.

The boy tossed the apple underhand across the room, which Doris caught. She had just sunk her teeth in the sweet apple when he suddenly belted out, "Hey everybody, look at the pig!"

All the guys turned toward Doris, who was frozen in mid-bite, which only accentuated the image of a pig roasting on a spit with an apple in its mouth. Laughter erupted, which mortified the teenager. Doris ran for her room, where she fell on her bed and bawled her eyes out the rest of the evening. She fell asleep weeping in misery.

"What that boy said that night has stuck with me all my life," she said. "I never had a good feeling about myself before that night, and I certainly didn't think very highly of myself after that."

It didn't help matters that Doris grew up as an Air Force brat, part of a family that moved every couple of years to the next posting. She always had a hard time making friends in places like Madrid and Aranjuez, Spain; Hamilton, Bermuda; Palermo, New Jersey; Seattle, Washington; and Ceres, California, a small central California town where she went to high school.

Eleven days after her high school graduation, she married the first person who showed an interest in her—Jack Williams, an Air Force aircraft electronic technician from Huntington, West Virginia. When their first son—named after his father—was born fifteen months later at their posting in the Philippines, Doris was tipping the scales at 235 pounds.

Jack, Jr. wasn't the only one gaining weight in those days. "I told friends that I was on the seafood diet: I would see food and eat it," Doris explained. "When we moved back to the States, I loved going to Perry Boy's, an all-you-can-eat restaurant, every Saturday night. I loved the variety of foods they served. I would skip the salad bar and fill up my plate with ham, bacon, fried chicken, mashed potatoes, and corn, making five or six trips through the buffet line." Her weight slowly but surely marched past 280 pounds after a second boy, Brian, was born.

Not only did Doris love to eat, but she loved to cook as well.

Her favorite recipe was one handed down from her mother—tacos from scratch, *muy authentico*. The recipe called for mixing ground beef with eggs, crushed saltine crackers or oatmeal, tomato paste or ketchup, and lots of crushed red peppers.

"I would take a golf-ball-sized piece of meat and place it in the middle of a corn tortilla," Doris explained. "Then I would smooth the meat out with my hand and fold the taco in half and place it in a pan filled with hot grease. After deep-frying the taco, I'd take it out, drain off the grease, open up the taco and put in a slice of Velveeta cheese, and go make the next one. For dinner, we'd add our own lettuce, tomato, onions, and avocados to the tacos. I would fix three dozen for the family and eat twelve or fifteen tacos in one sitting."

After twelve years of marriage, Doris and Jack divorced. She moved back to Central California and settled in Modesto, where she met and married Larry Bailey in 1982 while working as a certified nursing assistant in nursing and private homes. When her weight crept north of 300 pounds, she gave up hope of ever slimming down. Sure, she had tried the popular diets: Overeaters Anonymous, Jenny Craig, and Weight Watchers, but they never worked. "I would lose five pounds, but then I would overeat a little bit or not follow the diet to a T, and get six pounds back," she said. "That was really frustrating."

Then on a Sunday morning in early 2006, Doris was sitting with the congregation at Calvary Temple Worship Center in Modesto, minding her own business. I had been invited to minister at the morning services and shared a message about presenting our bodies as living sacrifices.

I challenged those in the audience that morning. "Can you say, 'This is the best I have, and I'm giving it to the Lord'?" I asked. "Are you an example of God's best? Can others see your vitality? Wouldn't it be awesome if God's people were so full of good health, so vibrant, that others would notice us from ten or twenty feet away?"

Doris didn't want to be noticed. She knew her health was far from vibrant. Decades of obesity had taken their toll: asthma, gout, osteoarthritis, acid reflux, high blood pressure, and sleep apnea. Her knees were shot: the only way she could walk was with the assistance of a cane or walker.

"I had never heard of you before you came to speak at my church," she told me. "When I heard you speak, I sat there in shock. The thing you said that made me open my eyes was when you urged us to eat only foods that God has created—not foods that man had created with terrible ingredients and additives or preservatives."

After I was done speaking that morning, one of the pastors, Kelli Williams, urged everyone in the church to attend weekly classes called the "7 Weeks of Wellness," which were based on the teachings found in my book, *The Great Physician's Rx for Health and Wellness*. The first class nailed it for Doris as she learned about Key #1: Eat to Live. Here's what happened in her own words:

> I went home and cleaned out my cupboards and refrigerator, and then I went shopping for foods that God created. I began eating many more salads and either

baked or broiled chicken. I stopped eating pork and sugary treats like jelly-filled doughnuts and apple turnovers. No more eating a half-gallon of ice cream in one sitting. I filled my refrigerator with fresh vegetables, organic whole milk, and even some goat's milk and goat's cheese, even though I wasn't too hip on that in the beginning. I ate apples, bananas, or oranges as my lunch.

I saw pounds immediately come off—and stay off. What a blessing for someone who had tried every diet for the last thirty-eight years with no sustained weight loss or health improvement until I tried the Great Physician's prescription. In a couple of months, I lost twenty-five pounds, going from 330 to 305 pounds!

God has given me the strength and ability to completely change the way I eat and live. I never knew that eating healthy and using portion control could do so much. After years of smorgasbords and fast food, now I cook fresh healthy foods at home. It's an adventure to cook healthy meals.

I'm encouraged to keep following what I have learned, and now I have given myself a new goal: to get down to 175 pounds by February 2009!

Taking a New Attitude

Doris Bailey has been following the Great Physician's prescription for health and wellness for less than three months now, and I wish her nothing but the best. She feels confident she can continue to lose weight because the Great Physician's prescription is not a diet but a whole new lifestyle. This attitude is more in line with the etymology of the word "diet," which originated from the Greek word *diaita*, meaning "life, lifestyle, way of living."

The fact that you're reading the *Great Physician's Rx for Weight Loss* tells me that losing weight is something you desire for yourself or for someone close to you. If so, you probably don't need to be reminded that packing on too many pounds is unhealthy or has become part of the national discussion these days. The evidence surrounds us when we're out in public: you would have to be Stevie Wonder not to notice all the jiggly tummies or padded thighs in the malls these days. As a culture, we are a little taller but a lot heavier than we were a generation ago; today we weigh twenty-five pounds more than our grandparents or parents did in the 1960s, with the biggest weight gains attached to men forty and older.

The latest National Center for Health statistics on overweight and obese people do not paint a rosy future for this country. An estimated 65 percent of U.S. adults aged twenty years and older weigh too much, which is defined as having a body mass index (BMI) of twenty-five or higher.

The body mass index is a mathematical formula that takes into account a person's height and weight and comes up with a corresponding number called the BMI. As a strict formula, the body mass index equals a person's weight in kilograms divided in height by meters squared. According to a body mass index table converted to pounds and inches for American use (these indexes are easily available online), the BMI breakdown goes like this:

- 18 or lower: underweight
- 19–24: normal
- 25–29: overweight
- 30–39: obese
- 40–54: extremely obese

As an example, someone standing five feet ten inches tall and weighing more than 209 pounds would have a BMI of 30, earning him or her a classification of obese on the body mass index scale. About 30 percent of the U.S. adult population has a BMI of 30 or more, which is remarkable.

As waistlines have expanded to Pillsbury Doughboy range, a sizable weight-loss industry has stepped into the vacuum, thanks to the insatiable appetite of more than 70 million Americans claiming to be on a diet at any one time. The U.S. weight-loss and diet control market could top $50 billion in 2006, according to Marketdata, a market research firm that has tracked diet products and programs since 1989. That works out to $136 million *a day* spent on the following:

- books promising the "newest" approach to weight loss, plus a handful of perennial bestsellers: *Atkins New Diet Revolution, South Beach Diet,* and *The Zone.*

- gastric bypass surgery, in which surgeons staple or bind the stomach with an adjustable band. This creates a small pouch able to hold only a few ounces of food. Celebrities such as singer Carnie Wilson and *Today Show* weatherman Al Roker sang the praises of this potentially dangerous surgery after shedding hundreds of pounds.

- commercial chains such as Weight Watchers, Jenny Craig, and LA Weight Loss, where dieters commit to structured programs. More than 7 million have signed up for these programs.

- over-the-counter diet pills such as CortiSlim and Trim Spa, which are heavily advertised on television and radio and target the lose-weight-quick crowd.

- diet food home delivery, where affluent dieters pay as much as $1,200 a month (per person!) for healthy meals to be delivered daily to their doorstep. A handful of companies such as Zone Chefs, NutriSystem, Seed Live Cuisine, and Jenny Direct (part of Jenny Craig) are cashing in on this booming market.

- weight-loss summer camps for heavy teens, which are a predictable outgrowth of the childhood obesity problem in this country. These types of camps didn't exist in my parents' time because the demand wasn't there. Today plump teens seek to turn their lives around at places like Camp La Jolla and Camp Shane.

For those who can't bear the thought of climbing aboard another diet train (after having experienced so much failure in the past), a host of entrepreneurial companies are marketing products promising to make life comfy and cushy for the overweight. WideBodies Furniture sells oversized sofas, love seats, and chairs.

LiftChair.com has introduced recliner chairs that lift and tilt forward so that morbidly obese people weighing as much as seven hundred pounds can get in and out of them more easily. For those who need a different type of seating, the Big John toilet seat is more receptive to an oversized tush: this toilet seat is a full five inches wider than the standard fourteen-inch-wide version.

Consumer research has helped huge corporations like GM and Ford tailor their products for Heavy America. The Detroit automakers have quietly widened seats in their SUVs and light pickup trucks so that heavyset drivers will have "plenty of leg room." You can scroll through Sizewise.com to determine which cars provide the most interior room, but some obese drivers have to take their cars into auto upholstery shops to have seatbelt extenders installed. Those who can't squeeze in behind the wheel have smaller steering wheels mounted at body shops.

Businesses are feeling the weight of heavier customers and employees. Airlines complain that their jets are burning more expensive fuel because passenger "payload" is heavier than ever. On the ground, large corporations and small businesses face skyrocketing medical insurance premiums because obese employees need more health care. Many HR departments are rearranging the office furniture to accommodate their employees' extra girth. Desk chairs that support five hundred pounds are being rolled into cubicles, while some businesses have had to install heavy-duty toilets (equipped with Big John toilet seats, I would imagine).

Hospitals, no doubt seeing more obese patients since overweight people are hospitalized more often than the general population, have installed patient hoists in certain rooms. They need the hoists on hand since orderlies cannot lift such large amounts of weight in and out of hospital beds without landing in the hospital themselves—with a hernia.

But these examples pale in comparison to an announcement in 2005 from a team of university researchers who stated that rising obesity rates could reverse life expectancy gains—the first time this has happened since the U.S. government began keeping track in 1900. Life expectancy in the United States is now at a high of 77.6 years, but according to a study published in the *New England Journal of Medicine*,[1] that could mean—and I have to emphasize the conditional here—that the generation of my toddler-aged son, Joshua, could live two to five years less.

What about you? I'm sure that you're aware that being overweight is a cause of high blood pressure, high cholesterol, hypertension, type 2 diabetes, and a host of other ailments that shorten one's life span.

And you're thinking something needs to be done.

CONVENTIONAL MEDICAL TREATMENT

Diet and exercise are often the first things prescribed by a physician when meeting with those needing to lose weight.

Of course. And snowbirds flock to Florida every winter. And there's a presidential election every four years.

But that advice falls on deaf ears, or the overweight patients give it their best only to fail for the umpteenth time. In subsequent visits, doctors will suggest that they go on a certain medication. That's what medical physicians have been trained to do:

make the diagnosis, fill out the prescription form, and send patients on their way.[2]

Giant pharmaceutical companies are pouring millions, if not billions, of research and development money into developing drugs that fight obesity. I wish them all the best, but I don't see a "weight loss" pill ever working, at least without sizable side effects. For those on the market today, the cure can be worse than the disease.

Some in the medical establishment are pinning their hopes on a new drug called Accomplia (also known by its pharmaceutical name, rimonabant), which works on a newly discovered system in the brain that is involved in the motivation and control of the appetite. FDA approval of rimonabant is expected in 2006, which will give physicians another weapon in their arsenal. Currently doctors prescribe two drugs for long-term obesity therapy—Xenical and Meridia. The former inhibits the absorption of fat in the stomach; the latter acts as an appetite suppressant. While the effectiveness of these drugs is open to debate, no one in modern medicine disputes that Xenical and Meridia have been traced to potentially serious side effects such as increased heart rate and long-term diarrhea. The Food and Drug Administration decided in 2005 not to ban Meridia despite reports of more than two dozen deaths and several hundred nonfatal strokes, heart attacks, and other cardiovascular ailments.

Since a doctor's advice to eat less and exercise more is usually ignored and the medical community lacks a "magic bullet" to prescribe with confidence, medical physicians are pointing obese patients toward a surgical option—gastric bypass surgery.

Since the late 1990s, gastric bypass surgeries have skyrocketed in response to demand. To keep pace, the number of doctors who have learned the surgical technique and joined the American Society for Bariatric Surgery has tripled since 2000. In addition, bariatric surgical centers are opening their doublewide doors in major cities around the country.

The development of laparoscopic surgical techniques has made the procedure much less invasive to the body. Gastric bypass surgeons staple the stomach—or bind it with an adjustable band—so that a small pouch is created to hold two or three ounces of food. This restricts food intake and interrupts the normal digestive process. People experience the sensation of being full after a few bites of food; if they eat any more, they often become nauseated. The idea is that obese patients will lose weight because they *can't* eat any more. A normal stomach holds eight to ten times more food.

Gastric bypass surgery is dangerous for your health because the odds of *not* surviving are higher than most patients realize, according to a recent Medicare study that analyzed the risks. A 2005 study that appeared in the *Journal of the American Medical Association* (*JAMA*) reported that more than 5 percent of men and nearly 3 percent of women ages thirty-five to forty-four were dead within a year of undergoing the surgery. Slightly higher mortality rates were discovered in patients forty-five to fifty-four. Among patients sixty-five to seventy-four years of age, 13 percent of men and 6 percent of women died. Wait, the news gets worse: male patients seventy-five years and older had a 50/50 chance of survival; female patients, a 40 percent chance.[3] Holy Toledo!

Another consideration is that gastric bypass surgery is expensive, costing around $25,000. Insurance companies, which have seen their bottom lines battered by hundreds of thousands of gastric bypass claims, are putting the kibosh on paying for any more gastric bypass procedures. Many patients have to come up with the money out-of-pocket or work out a payment plan with their doctors. And I feel compelled to point out that people with certain kinds of gastric bypass surgery have been known to let loose massive amounts of flatulence. That can hurt relationships.

The possibility of dying or having excessive gas hasn't slowed down the number of obese people marching into surgical centers. What started out as a radical option for the morbidly obese has become as routine as a dental office visit. More than 150,000 overweight people will submit to the scalpel in 2006, a huge leap from just 20,000 operations a decade ago. I understand the rationale behind these operations: these obese people have tried every diet known to man—and failed to keep the weight off.

Unfortunately between 5 and 20 percent of gastric bypass patients regain much or all of their weight after a few years. Having gastric bypass surgery is like using your last relief pitcher in a baseball game: there's no one left in the bullpen to call into the game. Once you shrink-wrap your stomach, you're out of medical options.

What's happening is that some gastric bypass patients learn to "outsmart" their fist-sized stomachs. They melt Hershey's chocolate in a sauce pan and sip the sweet concoction throughout the day, or they puree Dove Bars, grind up M&M's, or toss blueberry muffins in a blender with heavy cream.

When overweight people end up right back where they started, they feel like failures. In their minds, they messed up their last—and best—chance to lose weight and keep it off.

The Seven Truths About Obesity
by obesity specialist Gus Prosch Jr., M.D.

1. If you're obese, you have a lifetime disease.
2. Your metabolic processes will always tend to be abnormal.
3. You cannot eat what others eat and stay thin.
4. Anyone can lose weight and stay slim provided the causes of weight gain are determined, addressed, and corrected.
5. Understanding insulin metabolism is the key to losing weight intelligently.
6. There is absolutely no physiological requirement for sugar or processed foods in your diet.
7. You cannot lose weight and keep it off successfully by strictly and solely following any special diet, by taking a weight-loss pill, or by following an exercise program. To succeed, you must address all the contributing factors causing obesity. And you must make exercise and physical activity a lifetime effort.[4]

ALTERNATIVE MEDICAL TREATMENTS

At the other end of the spectrum are "alternative" approaches to weight loss. Certain herbs and herbal blends, such as *Garcinia cambogia,* are said to inhibit the conversion of excess calories to body fat. Glycogen, a stored form of glucose, is reputed to suppress the appetite. Nutritional products such as CellaFree, Cell Pill, and Cell-U-Lite are designed to battle cellulite, which is a series of fat cells and subcutaneous connective tissue rippling underneath the skin. These products reportedly help the body lose fat without losing lean muscle tissue.

The Natural Medicines Comprehensive Database lists more than 50 individual supplements and 125 proprietary products being marketed as weight-loss products, although their efficacy and long-term safety are question marks. Chromium, a popular weight-loss supplement, is found in many herbal blends. Guar gum, produced from Indian cluster beans, and chitosan, extracted from shellfish, are sold as "fat blockers."

In this country, dietary aids containing the herbal supplement ephedra were huge sellers until they were linked to 155 deaths, including Baltimore Orioles six-foot two-inch, 249-pound pitching prospect Steve Bechler in 2003. The U.S. Food and Drug Administration reacted by banning ephedra, but a federal judge threw out the FDA ban in 2005.

Ephedra was the main ingredient in herbal fen-phen, which was popular in the mid-1990s. Those seeking to lose weight back then were confused by the presence of an antiobesity drug called fen-phen, which was the combination of fenfluramine and phentermine. Takers of fen-phen (the drug), however, began experiencing disturbing side effects: manic depression, anxiety, and hallucinations. In 1997 the FDA forced the withdrawal of fen-phen from the market after numerous people came down with the disabling and potentially fatal disease of primary pulmonary hypertension.

Alternative medicine differs from conventional treatments in the area of nutritional supplements. Where medically trained physicians are more apt to prescribe a certain drug or popular diet, alternative medical publications such as *The Encyclopedia of Natural Healing* recommend daily dosages of vitamin B complex, lecithin, evening primrose oil, green food supplements, multimineral complex, and kelp.[5] Alternative medicine's justification for adding kelp and other exotic supplements is that overweight people tend to have poor nutritional intake and particularly low mineral and fatty acid levels. Evening primrose oil and flaxseed oil supply the body with essential fatty acids, which are needed for many body functions.

Adding enzymes to one's diet is another way to rev up metabolism and boost the immune system. *The Encyclopedia of Natural Healing* touts fresh, raw fruits for their enzyme-rich properties and commends cherries as a way to satisfy hunger urges. Cherries, which contain almost no calories from fat or protein, are great for metabolism, but *The Encyclopedia of Natural Healing* must *really* like cherries because the authors recommend eating three to five *pounds* a day. Careful: this might bring on an unforgettable case of the runs.

You should also be careful about wasting your hard-earned

money buying those electrical pads that you wrap around your stomach so that electrical stimulation can "burn" fat cells away. Companies pitching "fat burners" in late-night infomercials are no different from carnival barkers holding up a bottle of their snake oil, hoping to separate suckers from their cash.

Where We Go from Here

I teach a different approach to weight loss, which is based on the seven keys to unlock your God-given health potential found in my foundational book *The Great Physician's Rx for Health and Wellness:*

- Key #1: Eat to live.
- Key #2: Supplement your diet with whole food nutritionals, living nutrients, and superfoods.
- Key #3: Practice advanced hygiene.
- Key #4: Condition your body with exercise and body therapies.
- Key #5: Reduce toxins in your environment. Don't smoke cigarettes or use tobacco products.
- Key #6: Avoid deadly emotions.
- Key #7: Live a life of prayer and purpose.

Some of these keys, I admit, do not seem directly related to weight loss, but they are part of living a healthy lifestyle and will enable you to attain and maintain your ideal weight. I am convinced that you will lose extra pounds if you adopt these seven keys because I've met too many people and read too many e-mails from those who love telling me that they finally found a way to lose weight, get healthy, and live the life they've always dreamed of.

I believe each and every one of us has a God-given health potential that can be unlocked only with the right keys. I want to challenge you to incorporate these timeless principles and allow God to transform your health as you slash pounds and add years to your life.

KEY #1

Eat to Live

I would have loved hanging out with Benjamin Franklin if I were alive 250 years ago. When Ben was just twenty-seven years old, he published *Poor Richard's Almanack*, a compilation of weather reports, recipes, predictions, and opinions.

What got him noticed in the town square were his witty aphorisms and profound sayings, which would have made him a great blogger today. Here are a few of my favorites:

- "Work as if you were to live a hundred years, pray as if you were to die tomorrow."

- "Fish and visitors stink after three days."

- "Three may keep a secret, if two of them are dead."

Ben Franklin's wisdom—he was the first to suggest daylight saving time—is the reason why he became one of our founding fathers. But there's another Benjamin Franklin saying that I love, and it's the backbone of my first key. The Ben Franklin quote goes like this: "Eat to live, and not live to eat."

Satisfying hunger is said to be man's second-strongest urge, supplanted only by the desire to live. (If you thought it was sex, then you've been watching too many *Friends* reruns.) Since encountering truly life-threatening situations is about as rare as

1

winning a Powerball lottery these days, I believe the next primal urge—satisfying hunger—can loom larger than life these days. When you go without food for too long, gnawing hunger pangs create an almost overwhelming urge to satiate the appetite.

Physiologically speaking, hunger begins in the brain when the limbic system determines that the body is low in blood sugar. Hunger pangs can also come from a visual signal—watching an alluring TV advertisement promoting a grilled chicken panini sandwich, for instance. The thalamus in the limbic system converts the physical need into an urge, and depending on how hungry you become, that urge can range from "I think I'll snack on something" to "I'm hungry! I've got the munchies!"

Eventually this longing desire causes one to take physical steps to gratify the internal nagging to eat some food. When it comes to pleasing that urge, people follow the path of least resistance: they reach for something convenient—a microwavable meal prepared in conveyor-belt fashion at a far-away factory or a sack of fast food handed out a drive-through window. That's not the way you want to go through life, especially if you weigh too much.

I propose a new approach to weight loss, and it begins with my first key—"Eat to live." This principle involves choosing something to eat that will be better for your body in the long term rather than a quick fix to squelch hunger pangs. And in case you're concerned, healthy food can and often does taste great. I urge you to pay close attention because the foundation for the Great Physician's Rx for weight loss is being laid right here.

Memory Key

I have two principles—a pair of cornerstones—to lay on this foundation for weight loss. I won't guarantee that the pounds will melt away or that you'll lose four dress sizes, but if you follow these two vital concepts, you'll experience vibrant health and a slimmer physique.

Here they are:

1. Eat what God created for food.
2. Eat food in a form that is healthy for the body.

We can look to Scripture to be reminded about what God created for food. My friend, Rex Russell, M.D., compiled a comprehensive list of foods created by God in his book, *What the Bible Says About Healthy Living*. I've listed them here, along with the scriptural references:

- almonds (Gen. 43:11)
- barley (Judg. 7:13)
- beans (Ezek. 4:9)
- bread (1 Sam. 17:17)
- broth (Judg. 6:19)
- cakes (2 Sam. 13:8, and probably not the kind with frosting)
- cheese (Job 10:10)

- cucumbers, onions, leeks, melons, and garlic (Num. 11:5)
- curds of cow's milk (Deut. 32:14)
- figs (Num. 13:23)
- fish (Matt. 7:10)
- fowl (1 Kings 4:23)
- fruit (2 Sam. 16:2)
- game (Gen. 25:28)
- goat's milk (Prov. 27:27)
- grain (Ruth 2:14)
- grapes (Deut. 23:24)
- grasshoppers, locusts, and crickets (Lev. 11:22)
- herbs (Exod. 12:8)
- honey (Isa. 7:15) and wild honey (Ps. 19:10)
- lentils (Gen. 25:34)
- meal (Matt. 13:33)
- oil (Prov. 21:17)
- olives (Deut. 28:40)
- pistachio nuts (Gen. 43:11)
- pomegranates (Num. 13:23)
- quail (Num. 11:32)
- raisins (2 Sam. 16:1)
- salt (Job 6:6)
- sheep (Deut. 14:4)

- sheep's milk (Deut. 32:14)
- spices (Gen. 43:11)
- veal (Gen. 18:7–8)
- vegetables (Prov. 15:17)
- vinegar (Num. 6:3)[1]

Are any of these foods staples in your diet? Do you have to think hard to remember the last time you bit into a fresh apple, scooped up a handful of raisins, or supped on lentil soup? These listed foods are nutritional gold mines and contain no refined or processed carbohydrates and no artificial sweeteners. Since God has given us a wonderful array of natural foods to eat, it would take several pages to describe all the fantastic fruits and vibrant vegetables available from His garden. A diet based on consuming whole and natural foods harvested directly from the Creator's bounty fits within the bull's-eye of eating foods that God created in a form healthy for the body.

When it comes to losing weight, anyone who speaks with any credibility on the topic agrees that you will shed pounds if you do the following:

1. Consume fewer calories.

2. Increase caloric expenditure (exercise).

Eating God's foods in a form that He created is an instant way to consume fewer calories. According to the Mayo Clinic, you consume only sixty calories when you eat one of these foods as a snack:

- one small apple
- one-half cup of grapes
- two plums
- two tablespoons of raisins
- one and one-half cups of strawberries
- two cups of shredded lettuces
- one-half cup of diced tomatoes
- two cups of spinach
- three-fourths cup of green beans[2]

On the other hand, a Cold Stone Creamery treat—a medium-sized mocha ice cream with Reese's Pieces and Oreo cookies mixed in and topped with pistachio nuts—comes out to a whopping 1,150 calories, or *twice* the amount of calories contained in *all* the fruits and vegetables I just listed!

But, Jordan, if you're telling me to eat fruits and vegetables to lose weight, it can't be this simple. Well, just so you know, I'm not advocating a diet of low-cal fruits and vegetables, which does not provide the body with the full slate of nutrients that it needs, as I'll explain shortly. What I'm saying is that we're exiting ice-cream stores, fast-food restaurants, and supermarket checkout lines with processed foods pumped up with excess calories like baseball players on steroids. That's why we're having a nationwide problem with obesity.

LEADING OFF WITH NUTRIENTS

Our diets used to be pretty simple. We ate what was raised on the family farm or, if we lived in the city, what was *harvested* from the family farm—fruits; vegetables; wild grain and seeds; raw, unpasteurized dairy products; and meat from animals that grazed the fields. Wild game was obtainable, and since most major population centers were near an ocean or a waterway, fresh fish was readily available.

I believe God gave us physiologies that crave these foods in their natural state because our bodies are genetically set for certain nutritional requirements by our Creator. Our taste buds, however, have been manipulated by fast-food chains and restaurants that sweeten meats with secret sauces and top everything in sight with melted cheese and bacon. The strategy has worked: we've become a country that loves inexpensive, deep-fried, greasy food high in calories, high in fat, high in sugar, and—in most people's minds—high in taste. Taste trumps health, no matter how many calories or fat grams the food contains. This explains why fast-food chains and sit-down restaurants are purveyors of monster burgers, pail-sized barrels of fried chicken, and stuffed-crust pizza rising more than an inch high. When Denny's Beer Barrel Pub in Clearfield, Pennsylvania, announced that it was selling a 10.5-pound hamburger with twenty-five slices of cheese, columnist Bud Geracie of the *San Jose Mercury News* quipped, "And if you finish it, you get your name on a plaque—at the cemetery."[3]

We laugh, but it's no laughing matter how tens of millions each day queue up to purchase foods that are not in a form that

God created. Quick—how many times in the last week did you eat fast food? Two, three times? More?

Having an awareness of what you eat is an important first step to weight loss. As we begin traveling down this road together, I need to help you understand that everything you eat is a protein, a fat, or a carbohydrate. Each of these nutrients positively or negatively affects your weight and your entire body.

Let's take a closer look at these macronutrients.

THE FIRST WORD ON PROTEIN

Proteins, one of the basic components of foods, are the essential building blocks of the body. All proteins are combinations of twenty-two amino acids, which build body organs, muscles, and nerves, to name a few important duties. Among other things, proteins provide for the transport of nutrients, oxygen, and waste throughout the body and are required for the structure, function, and regulation of the body's cells, tissues, and organs.

Our bodies, however, cannot produce all twenty-two amino acids that we need to live a robust life. Scientists have discovered that eight essential amino acids are missing, meaning that they must come from other sources outside the body. Since we need these eight amino acids badly, it just so happens that animal protein—chicken, beef, lamb, dairy, eggs, and so on—is the only complete protein source providing the Big Eight amino acids. Better yet, eating protein supports weight loss.

We need the amino acids found in animal protein, and the best and most healthy sources are organically raised cattle, sheep, goats, buffalo, and venison. Grass-fed beef is leaner and lower in calories than grain-fed beef. Organic beef is higher in heart-friendly omega-3 fatty acids and important vitamins like vitamins B_{12} and E, and way better for you than assembly-line cuts of flank steak from hormone-injected cattle eating pesticide-sprayed feed laced with antibiotics.

Fish with scales and fins caught from oceans and rivers are lean sources of protein and provide the essential amino acids as well. Supermarkets are stocking these types of foods in greater quantities these days, and of course, they are found in natural food stores, fish markets, and specialty stores.

FAT CHANCE

If you've had a lifelong problem with being overweight, then you might approach fats in foods like a priest holding up a cross against a demon-possessed wild man. I wouldn't blame you for keeping fats at arm's length, especially if you were caught up in the low-fat craze from the mid-1990s. Back then, the conventional wisdom among diet books was that foods containing *any* fat were to be avoided. A generation of weight-conscious teen girls took that advice at face value, prompting an unprecedented leap in anorexia and bulimia. In their minds, fat was Public Enemy No. 1.

As it turned out, a diet of low-fat, reduced-fat, or fat-free foods didn't help anyone lose weight and keep it off. The problem with reduced-fat cookies and fat-free cream cheese was more than their low taste: these convenience foods had nearly the same amount of calories as the "full fat" versions. (And people would eat more fat-free cookies because they thought they could.)

There's a compelling reason why low-fat foods were not the hoped-for panacea. Chemically altering foods made things worse for the body, not better. God, in His infinite wisdom, created fats as a concentrated source of energy and source material for cell membranes and various hormones. Fats have a protective effect against heart disease.

People are often shocked to hear me say this, but this is why I say butter is better for you than margarine. The French understand my reasoning, and anyone who's vacationed in France with a red *Michelin Guide* in his or her hands has witnessed firsthand how the French diet is loaded with saturated fat in the form of butter, cheese, cream, meats, and rich pâtés like foie gras. Yet the French have a much lower rate of coronary heart disease than Americans, and deadly heart attacks claim half the victims in France as they do the United States. What we're learning from the French, says author Diana Schwarzbein of *The Schwarzbein Principle: The Truth About Losing Weight, Being Healthy, and Feeling Younger* (HCI, 1999), is that eating the right fats causes you to lose body fat and reach your ideal body composition.

Not all foods with fats deserve to be in your cupboard, however. Fats you want to steer away from are hydrogenated fats, which have been associated with a host of maladies, including diabetes, obesity, and cancer. Hydrogenated fats and partially hydrogenated fats are found in practically every processed food, from Dunkin' Donuts to Wonder Bread, from Ding Dongs to

Dove Bars. Most of the oils used in households today—soybean, safflower, cottonseed, and corn—are partially hydrogenated oils, which, by definition, are liquid fats that have been injected with hydrogen gas at high temperatures under high pressure to make them solid at room temperature.

Hydrogenation increases shelf life and gives flavor stability to foods, but it also produces unsaturated trans-fatty acids, also known as trans fat. Mark my words: trans fats are bad for you. Anything fried—chicken, steak, or fries—contains higher-than-average trans fat levels. For years, you couldn't find out how much trans fat was in the food you're eating, but that's changing in 2006 with the introduction of new Nutrition Facts labels stating the amount of trans fat in that particular food. I welcome this long-overdue change in food labeling.

Fats you want to include in your weight-loss regime are extra virgin coconut oil, extra virgin olive oil, and flaxseed oil, which are beneficial to the body and aid metabolism. I do not recommend that high-quality extra virgin olive oil be used in cooking, however, because certain nutrients in the olive oil break down when subjected to high heat. Use extra virgin coconut oil instead.

PICKING ON CARBOHYDRATES

Eating fat is not the reason why people get fat. Too many carbohydrates—especially those from refined sources—are often the culprits because the body has a limited capacity to store excess carbohydrates. Too much snacking, in a nutshell, forces the body to convert those excess carbohydrates into body fat.

A trio of low-carb weight-loss plans—Atkins, South Beach, and Zone—has been flying high for years. Their premise is that reducing the intake of carbohydrates like bread, pasta, and rice will reduce insulin levels and cause your body to burn excess body fat for fuel. The basic science behind the low-carb approach is this: reduce your intake of high-carbohydrate foods such as white flour and sugar, and increase your intake of high-protein sources, such as meat, fish, and dairy.

My biggest beef with low-carb diets is that most of these health plans call for a high consumption of meat products that God calls unclean (as I'll explain shortly), encourage the consumption of processed foods loaded with chemicals, recommend the use of artificial sweeteners, and allow a limited amount of nutrient-rich fruits and vegetables to be eaten.

Having said that, I believe in a lower carbohydrate approach to weight loss, and the carbohydrates you want to consume are low glycemic, high nutrient, and low in sugar. These would be found in fruits, vegetables, nuts, seeds, legumes, and cultured dairy products.

By definition, carbohydrates are the starches and sugars produced by plant foods. Starches and sugars, like fats, are not bad for you, but the problem is that the standard American diet is weighted way too heavily on the carbohydrate side, especially when you consider how many foods contain sugar. Sugar and its sweet relatives—corn syrup, fructose, sucrose, and maple syrup—are among the first ingredients listed in cereals, breads, buns, pastries, doughnuts, cookies, ketchup, and ice cream. Most people eat sugar with every meal: breakfast cereals are frosted with sugar, break time is soda or coffee mixed with sugar and a Danish, lunch has its cookies and treats, and dinner could be sweet-and-sour ribs, sweet potatoes, and corn on the cob, topped off with a sugary dessert. Talk about adding a sweet exclamation point to the day! A United States Department of Agriculture study in 2000 revealed that we eat an average of *thirty-two teaspoons* of sugar daily.

The other main carbohydrate form is starch, which is found in plant-based foods such as rice, potatoes, corn, and grains. When carbohydrates are eaten, the digestive tract breaks down the long chains of starches into single sugars, mainly glucose, which is a source of immediate energy. If these calories are not expended, the body converts them to fat, and therein lies a weighty problem.

You can't lose weight and keep it off when your diet is defined by too many *refined* carbohydrates. Refined foods will never match up to the nutritional power of fresh fruits and vegetables. The refining process strips grains, vegetables, and fruits of their vital fiber, vitamins, and mineral components.

The Great Physician's Rx for weight loss calls for eating your carbohydrates fresh and unrefined. This includes large amounts of fruits and vegetables, properly prepared grains and dairy products, nuts, seeds, legumes, and small amounts of honey and other healthy sweeteners.

FIBER IS FINE

Fiber is the indigestible remnant of plant cells found in vegetables, fruits, whole grains, nuts, seeds, and beans. Fiber-rich foods work their way through the digestive tract slowly, absorbing water and increasing the elimination of waste matter in the large intestine. This gives you an urge to have a bowel movement. Without fiber in your diet, you literally walk around feeling "down in the dumps" from constipation.

Fiber helps with weight loss by satisfying your hunger so that you're not tempted to fill up on fatty and sugary foods. Good sources of fiber are nuts; seeds; beans; whole grain sprouted breads; whole grains such as quinoa, amaranth, buckwheat, millet, and brown rice; green peas; carrots; cucumbers; zucchini; tomatoes; and baked or boiled unpeeled potatoes. Green leafy vegetables like spinach and fresh fruit are also fiber rich.

You also need to chew your food well. If people tease you about "inhaling" your food, then you're eating too fast. I recommend chewing each mouthful of food twenty-five to seventy-five times before swallowing. I know this sounds ridiculous, but if you chew your food longer, the brain will receive a signal that you're getting full, so you feel satiated earlier. Chewing slowly and thoroughly can help maintain a healthy weight as you allow your brain to register the amount of food you are consuming. Put simply, people who chew more consciously eat less and experience fewer digestive problems. Another way to feel full without eating as much as before is to eat nuts, seeds, and nut and seed butters, which contain fats that buffer insulin spikes and tell the brain that the stomach is feeling full.

Eat, Cheat, and Be Healthy?

Let's say you're invited to a Super Bowl party. Tables are piled high with tantalizing hors d'oeuvres, crispy finger foods, and tempting sweets. You indulge. You graze. You keep on eating. You're cheating.

How can you minimize the damage? According to Richard and Rachael Heller, authors of *The Carbohydrate Addict's Diet* (Signet, 1993), if you're going to cheat, then get it over with in a one-hour time frame. The Hellers say that when the body has been deprived of insulin-releasing foods high in carbohydrates, the body makes an adjustment. In other words, when you eat during one sixty-minute time frame, the body can be triggered to produce only so much insulin. Continue to snack longer—like right into the second half of the big game—and the body releases a second phase of insulin.

The Hellers advise that when you know you'll be put in a situation that may sabotage your weight-loss plans, make sure you eat a healthy low-carb breakfast and lunch loaded with healthy protein, fat, fruit, and vegetables. Then when you're with friends at a Super Bowl party, notice what time you go through the buffet line—and limit yourself to eating for sixty minutes. Be sure to avoid consuming any of what I call the Dirty Dozen foods (see the list on page 20). Get used to listening to your body—and noting how full you feel—whether you're foraging past a table of alluring foods or eating by yourself on the road.

In addition to the urge to cheat, you have to deal with food cravings. More often than not, those trying to lose weight suddenly crave foods that are verboten, prompting them to wistfully say, "Losing weight would be easy if the cravings would stop." An efficient way to dampen cravings is to eat foods that aid the body's production of serotonin, a neurotransmitter that gives you a feeling of well-being. Foods known to help the body produce serotonin are cottage cheese, milk, cheese, chicken, turkey, duck, and sesame seeds.

NUTRITION IN A BAR

In an effort to eat healthy and lose weight, many Americans have turned to consuming energy bars as a convenient meal replacement or as an in-between snack. This may sound like a good idea, but in reality, many energy bars are no healthier than a Snickers candy bar. In fact, many energy bars contain harmful ingredients such as artificial sweeteners, chemicals, preservatives, and synthetic nutrients.

The answer is eating a healthy whole food bar containing the highest quality protein, carbohydrates, fats, and fiber, as well as vitamins, minerals, probiotics, and enzymes. In my quest for providing others with healthy alternatives, I've developed one of the finest organic whole food bars available today, containing recommended amounts of protein, omega-3 fats, fiber, and probiotics, along with compounds known as beta-glucans from soluble oat fiber. If you find it difficult to pack a lunch or you frequent the vending machines during snack breaks—or you are searching for a healthy after-school treat for the kids—then check out these whole food bars. (For more information, visit www.BiblicalHealthInstitute.com and click on the GPRx Resource Guide.)

THE TOP HEALING FOODS

We have discussed many healthy foods in this chapter so far, but including the following foods in your diet is a must. In addition, keep this in mind when you sit down to eat: you should consume the proteins, fats, and vegetables first before swallowing any fruit, sweeteners, or high-starch carbohydrates like potatoes, rice, grains, and bread. I know it's hard to resist fresh bread when it's presented in a nice restaurant, but you would be better off having a piece toward the end of your entrée. (Maybe by then, you'll be so full that you can pass on this carbohydrate-rich food.)

1. Wild-Caught Fish
Fish caught in the wild are a richer source of omega-3 fats, protein, potassium, vitamins, and minerals than farm-raised fish, which are kept in cement ponds and fed a diet of food pellets. You can purchase fresh salmon and other wild-caught fish from your local fish market or health food store. Many other fish are healthy as well, including sardines, herring, mackerel, tuna, snapper, bass, and cod.

2. Cultured Dairy Products from Goats, Cows, and Sheep
Dairy products derived from goat's milk and sheep's milk can be healthier for some individuals than those from cows,

although dairy products from organic or grass-fed cows can be excellent as well. Goat's milk is less allergenic because it does not contain the same complex proteins found in cow's milk.

I do not recommend drinking 2 percent or skim milk because removing the fat makes the milk less nutritious and less digestible, and can cause allergies. Yes, whole milk has more calories, but this is not an area to cut corners. I've seen research suggesting that the mix of nutrients found in milk, such as calcium and protein, may improve the body's ability to burn fat, particularly around the midsection.

3. A Wide Selection of Fruits and Vegetables

Nutritionists have long known that fruits and vegetables are low in calories and high in fiber content. As mentioned earlier, eating plenty of fruits and vegetables—five servings a day are recommended—benefits those wanting to lose weight.

I've described how fruits and vegetables satisfy your hunger with fewer calories. You're going to save hundreds of calories a day by substituting sweets with just-as-sweet in-season fruits. Many fruits and vegetables are high in water, which provides volume in the pit of your stomach, not calories. Since these high-fiber foods take longer to digest, you feel full longer. It's kind of like having gastric bypass surgery without all the nasty side effects.

4. Soaked and Sprouted Seeds and Grains

Like fruits and vegetables, sprouted grains, seeds, nuts, and whole grains are higher in fiber. *Whole grain* means the bran and germ are left on the grain during processing. *Soaked grains* retain their plant enzymes when they are not cooked. This process greatly helps digestion.

5. Cultured and Fermented Vegetables

Often greeted with upturned noses at the dinner table, fermented vegetables such as sauerkraut, pickled carrots, beets, or cucumbers are overlooked by those on a diet, even though they are some of the healthiest foods on the planet. Raw cultured or fermented vegetables supply the body with useful organisms known as probiotics, as well as many vitamins, including vitamin C.

If you've never put a fork on any of these foods before, I urge you to sample sauerkraut or pickled beets, which are readily available in health food stores.

6. Healthy Fats

Foods high in healthy fats—olives, avocados, nuts and seeds and their butters, olive oil, flaxseed oil, coconut oil, and butter—can be wonderful allies in your quest for weight loss. Extra virgin coconut oil has been the recipient of some great press the last few years for its ability to help balance the thyroid, aid in metabolism, and help the body with energy production. Some experts recommend that people with thyroid and weight troubles should consume as many as two to four tablespoons of coconut oil per day. Make sure you consume healthy fats with every meal to provide satiety and slow the absorption of sugar into the bloodstream, thereby keeping blood sugar and insulin levels on an even keel.

A balanced thyroid plays a vital role in your metabolism. Mary Shomon, author of *The Thyroid Diet*, says that certain foods high in tyrosine assist the body in the production of the thyroid hormone, T3, which helps you utilize more oxygen and burn more calories. Foods high in tyrosine are cottage cheese, egg whites, safflower seeds, and meats such as turkey, antelope, quail, and buffalo.

7. Herbs and Spices

The use of herbs (rather than rich sauces on meats) and spices (rather than dressings, creams, or oil) is an excellent strategy for weight loss. I'm not talking about dousing your food with table salt, which is high in sodium, but reaching for strong flavors such as garlic, chili powder, cayenne, curry powder, rosemary, and tarragon to add taste to the foods you eat.

If you're following my advice to increase your eating of vegetables, douse them with lemon juice or spice them with basil and cilantro.

RUN, DON'T WALK, AWAY FROM THESE FOODS

Whether you have ten pounds or one hundred pounds to lose, certain foods should never find a way onto your plate or into your hands. Here are my Dirty Dozen, followed by a short commentary:

1. *Pork products.* In all of my books, I've consistently pointed out that pork—America's "other white meat"—should be avoided because pigs were called "unclean" in Leviticus and Exodus. God

labeled certain animals, birds, and fish "unclean" because they are scavengers who feed off trash—or worse.

2. *Shellfish and fish without fins and scales, such as catfish, shark, and eel.* God called hard-shelled crustaceans such as lobsters, crabs, and clams unclean as well in the Old Testament. Their flesh harbors known toxins that can contribute to poor health.

3. *Hydrogenated oils.* Margarine and shortening are taboo.

4. *Artificial sweeteners.* Aspartame, saccharin, sucralose, and its sweet cousins are made from chemicals that have sparked debate for decades. In addition, there is no proof that these noncaloric sweeteners improve metabolism; in fact, the opposite may be true.

5. *White flour.* One thing we've learned over the years: enriched white flour is not a dieter's best friend.

6. *White sugar.* If you're looking for a culprit to blame for bellies hanging over beltlines, then look no further.

7. *Soft drinks.* These are nothing more than liquefied sugar. A twelve-ounce can of Coke or Pepsi is the equivalent of eating nearly nine teaspoons of sugar.

8. *Pasteurized homogenized skim milk.* Like I said, whole organic milk is better, and goat's milk is best.

9. *Corn syrup.* This version of sugar is even more fattening.

10. *Hydrolyzed soy protein.* If you're wondering what in the world this is, hydrolyzed soy protein is found in imitation meat products. Stick to the real stuff.

11. *Artificial flavors and colors.* These are never good for you under the best of circumstances, and certainly not when you're trying to lose weight.

12. *Excessive alcohol.* Although studies point out the benefits of drinking small amounts of red wine for the heart—known as the "French Paradox"—the fact remains that alcohol contains lots of calories. Overconsumption of alcohol has wrecked millions of families over the years.

WHAT ABOUT FASTING?

Although skipping meals has proven not to lead to sustained weight loss, I do recommend giving the body a break by fasting once a week. Not only will your physical health improve, but there are spiritual benefits to be gained.

I believe a partial, one-day fast once a week—missing breakfast and lunch before eating dinner that night—will help you feel great and help you lose weight since you're eating less calories that week. I usually fast on Thursdays or Fridays since it's difficult to fast on weekends. If you've never voluntarily fasted for a day, give it a try and see how your body reacts. Be sure to drink plenty of water or raw juices, since these liquids do not require the digestive system to work hard while it rests and repairs.

THE IMPORTANCE OF HYDRATION

Drinking plenty of water is also important when you're *not* fasting. Water performs many vital tasks for the body: regulating the body temperature, carrying nutrients and oxygen to the cells, cushioning joints, protecting organs and tissues, and removing toxins. Water happens to be the perfect fluid replacement; only

God could come up with a calorie-free and sugar-free substance that makes up 92 percent of blood plasma and 50 percent of everything else in the body. The problem is that people don't drink enough water, or the liquids they sip contain so many calories—like a grande Mint Mocha Chip Frappuccino with 530 calories.

Every diet book worth its salt—I hope saying "salt" is making you thirsty—encourages readers to "drink eight glasses of water each day." This advice to drink water is overlooked by many seeking to lose weight, however, because they aren't aware that drinking fluids will put a damper on the hunger pangs coming from the pit of their stomachs. Downing a glass of water a half hour before lunch or dinner will act like a governor on an engine, taking the edge off your hunger pangs and preventing you from raiding the fridge or pillaging the pantry.

F. Batmanghelidj, M.D. and author of *You're Not Sick, You're Thirsty!*, contends that you will lose weight if you drink a glass of water one-half hour before you eat and two glasses two and a half hours later. "You will feel full and will eat only when food is needed," he says. "The volume of food intake will decrease drastically. The type of cravings for food will also change. With sufficient water intake, we tend to crave proteins more than carbohydrates. If you think you are different and your body does not need eight to ten glasses of water each day, you are making a major mistake," notes Dr. Batmanghelidj,[4] who believes that many dieters confuse hunger and thirst, thinking they're hungry when actually they're dehydrated.

Try to drink at least eight glasses of water, even if you

have to force yourself to swallow so much liquid. Sure, you'll go to the bathroom more often, but is that so bad? Drinking plenty of water is not only healthy for the body, but it's a key part of the Great Physician's Rx for Weight Loss Battle Plan (see page 74), so keep a water bottle close by and drink water before meals.

COFFEE BREAK

Speaking of something to drink, is this country's obsession with Starbucks coffee healthy? Many health experts disagree about whether consuming caffeinated beverages such as coffee or tea is a good idea, but I must point out that coffee and tea have been consumed for thousands of years by some of the world's healthiest people. Although I'm not a huge fan of coffee or a coffee drinker myself, I will say that fresh ground organic coffee flavored with organic cream and honey is fine when consumed in moderation, meaning one cup per day. Teas and herbal infusions (the latter beverage is made from herbs and spices rather than the actual tea plant) are another story all together.

Infusions of herbs and spices such as teas have been a part of nearly every culture throughout history. In fact, consuming organic teas and herbal infusions several times per day can be one of the best things you can do for your health. Green and white teas, for example, provide the body with antioxidants such as polyphenols, which help reduce cellular damage and oxidative stress. Studies have identified the anticancer compounds in tea as well as compounds that help increase metabolism. Teas and herbal infusions can provide energy, enhance the immune system, improve the digestion, and even help you wind down after a long day.

As far as caffeine is concerned, I believe that teas' benefits are better delivered in teas containing caffeine. Since tea leaves naturally contain caffeine, the Creator obviously intended for us to consume tea in its most natural form. Obviously, if caffeine tends to keep you up at night, you should avoid consuming caffeinated teas in the late afternoon or in the evening. For an after-dinner treat, try consuming a caffeine-free herbal infusion containing relaxing herbs and spices to help you wind down and decompress.

My favorite tea blends contain combinations of tea (green, black, or white) with biblical herbs and spices such as grape, pomegranate, hyssop, olive, and fig leaves. Even though I've never thought of myself as a tea-drinking type, my wife, Nicki, and I enjoy these biblical tea blends with dinner.

You'll find in my Great Physician's Rx for Weight Loss Battle Plan (see page 74) that I recommend a cup of hot tea and honey with breakfast, dinner, and snacks. I also advise consuming freshly-brewed iced tea, as tea can be consumed hot or steeped and iced. Please note that while herbal tea provides many great health benefits, nothing can replace pure water for hydration. Although you can safely and healthfully consume two to four cups per day of tea and herbal infusions, you still need to drink at least six cups of pure water for all the good reasons I've described in this chapter.

EAT: What Foods Are Extraordinary, Average, or Trouble?

I've prepared a comprehensive list of foods that are ranked in descending order based on their health-giving qualities. For a listing of Extraordinary, Average, and Trouble Foods, visit www. BiblicalHealthInstitute.com/EAT. Foods at the top of the list are healthier than those at the bottom. When eating, practice portion control. Put less food on your plate than you usually do, and see how it goes. A Pennsylvania State University study found that reducing serving size by 25 percent can help you consume up to eight hundred fewer calories per day without reducing satisfaction.[5]

The best foods to serve and eat are what I call Extraordinary, which God created for us to eat and are in a form healthy for the body. If you are struggling with your weight, it is best to consume foods from the Extraordinary category more than 75 percent of the time.

Foods in the Average category should make up less then 50 percent of your daily diet. If you are struggling with your weight, it's best to limit consumption of average foods to less than 25 percent of your daily diet.

Foods in the Trouble category do not promote weight loss and should be consumed with extreme caution. If you are trying to lose weight, you should avoid these foods completely.

℞ THE GREAT PHYSICIAN'S Rx FOR WEIGHT LOSS: EAT TO LIVE

- *Eat only foods God created.*

- *Eat foods in a form healthy for the body.*

- *At mealtime consume protein, fat, and veggies before starchy carbohydrates.*

- *Practice portion control by putting 25 percent less on your plate.*

- *Drink six to eight or more glasses of pure water per day and drink eight ounces of water whenever you feel hungry.*

- *When the plate is half-eaten, take a deep breath and ask yourself if you're still hungry.*

- *Partially fast one day per week.*

- *Chew each mouthful of food twenty-five to seventy-five times.*

- *Drink teas regularly.*

- *Consume whole food bars with one and one-half to three grams of beta-glucans from soluble oat fiber per day.*

Take Action

To learn how to incorporate the principles of eating to live, please turn to page 74 for the Great Physician's Rx for Weight Loss Battle Plan.

KEY #2

Supplement Your Diet with Whole Food
Nutritionals, Living Nutrients, and Superfoods

One reason I like shopping in natural food stores is the absence of tabloids at the checkout stands. When I do catch some headlines at an airport kiosk, I wonder where they come up with this stuff:

- "Earwax DNA Doesn't Lie: Osama Bin Laden Is a Woman!"
- "Hairy Space Alien Lives on Donald Trump's Head!"
- "Guy Calls Phone # on Toilet Wall—& Finds His Missing Mom!"

Listen, we can all enjoy a laugh, but what isn't funny is what's inside the tabloids, where over-the-top ads promise quick, easy weight loss. These quarter-page ads usually include a blurred photo of a flabby, unhappy woman juxtaposed next to a buff, slimmed-down version who looks vaguely familiar to the Ugly Duckling in the first panel.

"No Diet or Exercise Required!" blares the headline. If you've been looking for a way to finally "take it off and keep it off," then all you have to do is gulp down the $39.95 "all-natural dietary supplements" three times a day and watch the fat melt away.

Weight-loss pills have been advertised since the nation's first tabloid, the *Police Gazette,* was sold a hundred years ago. Back then, weight-loss drugs often contained laxatives (that'll make you lose weight) or synthetic insecticides to purportedly increase human metabolism. These diet potions usually worked for a while—if they didn't cause the runs, blindness, or some other major health catastrophe.

If you're trying to lose weight, I think you should take something *far* different from diet pills. I'm referring to whole food nutritional supplements and superfoods such as an organic green/whole food fiber blend, which can ensure the body an adequate supply of essential nutrients and beneficial compounds as one takes small steps toward weight loss.

LEADING OFF WITH MULTIVITAMINS

Believe it or not, many overweight and obese people are starved of nutrients because their diets contain mostly "empty" calorie foods. If you are among the majority of Americans who begin each day by gulping a multivitamin or two with your orange juice, I have a question for you: Have you checked the label of your multivitamin lately? If you see ingredients such as sucrose, corn starch, thiamine mononitrate, pyridoxine hydrochloride, or sodium metasilicate listed, your multivitamin is produced from isolated and synthetic materials.

Synthetic multivitamins are never going to be as good or potent as ones produced from natural sources; studies show that synthetically made vitamins are 50 to 70 percent less biologically active than vitamins made from natural sources. Another give-away is seeing the letters *dl* in front of an ingredient. An ingredient named "dl-alpha tocopheryl," for example, informs you that you're taking a synthetic version of vitamin E.

Since the body does not absorb more than 50 percent of the vitamins and minerals you ingest—you can see that in the way your urine changes to a fluorescent yellow—that means you're receiving only 25 percent of the advertised potency from chemically produced multivitamins. Take a whole food natural source multivitamin, which will double the nutrients absorbed by the body.

OMEGA-3 COD-LIVER OIL

Yes, most people turn up their noses at the thought of sipping a teaspoon of this fishy-smelling liquid, but they shouldn't. Any connection between weight loss and high omega-3 cod-liver oil (or fish oil) is anecdotal, but I've been taking cod-liver oil daily for the better part of ten years and greatly believe in its health-giving properties. After all, fishing communities in the North Atlantic countries of Norway, Scotland, and Iceland discovered the health benefits of cod-liver oil during the nineteenth century. Cod-liver oil was commonly given to ward off rickets in malnourished children, and its vitamin D helped build strong bones. The omega-3 fats contained in cod-liver or fish oil can improve cardiovascular health and help balance insulin levels.

Cod-liver oil is a superstar because it contains four nutrients that we hardly get enough of: eicosapentaenoic acid (EPA) and docosahexaenoic acid (DHA), vitamin A, and vitamin D. EPA and DHA are long-chain polyunsaturated fats known as omega-3 fatty acids, which are found in cold-water fish and eggs from chickens that run around and eat worms. The omega-3 fatty acids are wonderful not only for your immune system, but also for your skin health. Cod-liver oil contains more vitamin A per unit weight than other common foods, and its high levels of vitamin D are helpful if you're trying not to get too much sun.

Don't let the fishy taste keep you from introducing this nutrient into your diet. These days, cod-liver oil comes in lemon mint and other flavors that mask the odor and taste; for the less daring, omega-3 cod-liver oil comes in easy-to-swallow liquid capsules.

GREEN SUPERFOODS

"Eat your vegetables, or you don't get dessert."

How many times did you hear Mom or Dad say that? So you grudgingly stuffed a few green beans in your mouth and managed to get them down the hatch.

The dislike of eating vegetables, especially green vegetables, follows many people into adulthood. They know that they *should* eat more vegetables, but they regard salads and vegetable servings as colorful decorations for the main event—the meat and potatoes. Many people feel this way: the United States Department of Agriculture estimates that more than 90 percent of the U.S. population fails to eat the recommended three to five servings of vegetables each day.

You're not going to lose weight if you eschew your vegetables, especially the most beneficial—deep green leafy vegetables. You don't have much excuse: a modern transportation system delivers fresh salads and vegetables into every nook and cranny of our land.

Green foods are important for those losing weight because a lower carbohydrate diet means that you may not be getting all the vegetables and nutrients you need. Green foods will plug that gap.

Now there's a way to get your green foods that works great for those seeking to lose weight. It's through the consumption of green superfood powders and caplets, which are an excellent and easy way to receive the vitamins, minerals, antioxidants, and enzymes found in green leafy vegetables. All you do is mix green superfood powder in water or juice, or you can choose to swallow a handful of caplets.

A quality green food supplement is a certified organic blend of dried green vegetables, fermented vegetables, sea vegetables, microalgaes such as spirulina and chlorella, and sprouted grains and seeds. If you mix a couple of scoops of green food powder into a glass of water or juice, you'll be drinking one of the most nutrient-dense foods on this green earth—and receiving less than one-twentieth the calories of a Big Mac value meal!

This is what I call a real two-fer: not only is a green food supplement high in nutrients and low in calories, but it gives you the dietary benefits of whole food living nutrients, including keeping you as regular as the Swiss train system.

WHOLE FOOD FIBER BLEND

As mentioned in Key #1, fiber can be one of a dieter's best friends. Consuming adequate fiber ensures a feeling of satiety as fiber delays the absorption of sugars in the body and provides a sense of fullness. Fiber improves regularity, which helps to efficiently eliminate toxins from the body. Unfortunately most of us get about one-fifth of the optimal amount of fiber in our daily diet, which is why I recommend taking a whole food fiber supplement. Look for one that supplies your body with a highly usable, vegetarian source of dietary fiber.

Be sure to choose a brand made from organic seeds, grains, and legumes that are fermented or sprouted for ease of digestion. One of the best ways to consume whole food fiber is by taking a combination green superfood/fiber blend first thing in the morning and just before bed. Just mix it with your favorite juice or water, and you're giving your body more nutrition than most people get that day—or perhaps that week. Look for a green food fiber blend containing beta-glucans from soluble oat fiber, which can aid in providing satiety for the body and promoting a healthy body weight. (For a list of recommended whole food fiber products, visit www.BiblicalHealthInstitute.com and click on the GPRx Resource Guide.)

ENZYMES

If you're overweight, you've probably experienced your share of digestive problems. When you eat raw foods such as salads and fruits, you consume the enzymes they contain. When you eat cooked or processed meals, like those you get in a restaurant, however, the body's pancreas must produce the enzymes necessary to digest the meal. The constant demand for enzymes strains the pancreas, which must kick in more enzymes to keep up with the demand. Without receiving the proper levels of enzymes from raw or fermented foods—or from taking supplements—you are susceptible to excessive gas and bloating, constipation, heartburn, and low energy.

Digestive enzymes are complex proteins involved in the digestive process. They are the body's day laborers, the ones responsible for synthesizing, delivering, and eliminating the unbelievable number of ingredients and chemicals that your body uses during the waking hours. When the body produces enzymes, their job is to stimulate chemical changes in the foods passing through the gut. As mentioned before, the pancreas takes the lead role in producing digestive enzymes for the body.

Those with pancreatic problems such as cystic fibrosis usually require some form of digestive enzyme, but junk food diets, fast chewing, and eating on the run contribute to the body's inability to produce adequate enzyme production and the subsequent malabsorption of food. These problems worsen as you age.

If you're having trouble finding a way to eat enough raw, fresh foods such as bananas, avocados, seeds, nuts, grapes, and other natural foods, take plant-based digestive enzymes to ease food digestion. (You can find recommended brands by visiting www.BiblicalHealthInstitute.com and clicking on the GPRx Resource Guide.)

PROTEIN POWDER

I recommend the supplemental use of protein powders because protein definitely has a fat-burning effect on the body. Protein provides other benefits as well by reducing hunger (which hopefully stops you from consuming more calories) and helping to preserve muscles as those pounds drop off.

Commercially made protein powder is not as healthy as it may seem since it's usually derived from soy, milk, or whey protein. Most protein powders are highly processed and derived from cows injected with hormones and fed antibiotic grain or from genetically modified soybeans. You'll find many whey- or soy-based protein powders contain artificial sweeteners, flavorings, and additives.

The healthier option is choosing whey protein powders from grass-fed, free-range cows, fermented soy protein, or protein powder made from goat's milk. These are foods that God created in a form healthy for the body.

MEAL REPLACEMENT POWDERS

People who need to lose a lot of weight sometimes go on liquid diets, mixing a meal replacement powder in water to receive sustenance. Nick Yphantides, a San Diego physician whom I met, described how he lost more than 250 pounds (after weighing 467 pounds to begin with) over a nine-month period in his compelling book, *My Big Fat Greek Diet* (Nelson Books, 2004).

If you choose to try the same approach, be careful in your

selection of meal replacement powder, and those seeking to lose megaweight like Dr. Nick should only do so under a doctor's supervision. If you proceed, I recommend a meal replacement powder that contains easily digestible protein, beta-glucans from soluble oat fiber, organic fruits, sprouted seeds, live probiotics, omega-3 fatty acids, and antioxidants. (For recommended products, visit www.BiblicalHealthInstitute.com and click on the GPRx Resource Guide.)

 THE GREAT PHYSICIAN'S Rx FOR WEIGHT LOSS: SUPPLEMENT YOUR DIET

- *Take a whole food living multivitamin with each meal.*

- *Consume one-to-three teaspoons or three-to-nine capsules of high omega-3 cod-liver oil (or fish oil) per day with dinner.*

- *Each morning and before bedtime, take a serving of a green food/fiber blend.*

- *To improve digestion, take a probiotic/enzyme formula with each meal.*

- *Consume one capsule of a herbal adaptogen/antioxidant blend with each meal.*

- *To ensure optimal protein intake, incorporate an easily digestible protein powder into your daily diet.*

Take Action

To learn how to incorporate the principles of supplementing your diet with whole food nutritionals, living nutrients, and superfoods, please turn to page 74 for the Great Physician's Rx for Weight Loss Battle Plan.

KEY #3

Practice Advanced Hygiene

I will be the first to admit that dipping your face into a basin of facial solution, cleaning under your fingernails with a special soap, and washing your hands after going to the bathroom don't sound as if they have much to do with losing weight.

But there's an aspect of good hygiene that's relevant to this discussion, and it's the important role of the immune system in your body. Your immune system, which is ultrasensitive to changes in the body's defense capabilities, is negatively impacted by yo-yo dieting, according to research at the Fred Hutchinson Cancer Research Center. Repeatedly losing weight—only to regain it—apparently influences natural-killer-cell activity in the immune system. Known as NK cells, these cells are a vital line of defense for the body's immune system because they kill viruses as well as cancer cells, according to laboratory tests. The way I see it, your body will better protect you from life-threatening diseases like cancer if you lose weight and keep it off, and you'll be even *more* protected if you're the cleanest dieter on the block.

As I said, there isn't a direct link between practicing advanced hygiene and weight loss, but you'll be better off by incorporating this aspect of the Great Physician's Rx for health and wellness into your life.

CLEAN PRINCIPLES

What do I mean by the phrase "advanced hygiene"?

I'm glad you asked because I'm a great believer in protecting myself from harmful germs, and I've been practicing an advanced hygiene protocol for more than a decade. I've witnessed the results in my own life: no lingering head colds, no nagging sinus infections, and no acute respiratory illnesses to speak of for many years.

I follow a program first developed by an Australian scientist, Kenneth Seaton, Ph.D., who discovered that ear, nose, throat, and skin problems could be linked to the fact that humans touch the nose, eyes, and mouth with germ-carrying fingernails throughout the day.

In scientific terms, this is known as auto- or self-inoculation. So how do your fingernails get dirty?

Through hand-to-hand contact with surfaces and other people. If you thought that most germs were spread by airborne exposure—someone sneezing at your table—you would be wrong. "Germs don't fly; they hitchhike," Dr. Seaton declared, and he's right.

Dr. Seaton estimates that once you pick up hitchhiking germs, they hibernate and hide around the fingernails, no matter how short you keep them trimmed. You would be surprised to find out how much you scratch your nose or rub your mouth and eyes; but if you're like most people, it's a constant habit. When you come into contact with contagious germs, you can get sick, come down with the common cold, or find yourself battling the flu. This happens all the time. Chuck Gerba, a University of

Arizona environmental-microbiology professor, says that 80 percent of infections, from cold and flu viruses to food-borne diseases, are spread through contact with hands and surfaces.

How do you get germs on your hands? By shaking hands with others or touching things they touched: handrails, doorknobs, shopping carts, paper money, coins, and food. That last one—food—is a big one. You may remember reading about the Norwalk virus, which was blamed for a rash of illnesses on cruise ships in recent years. According to the Centers for Disease Control and Prevention, the only source of the Norwalk virus was feces from infected people, meaning that people who were tossing salads and handling food in the ship's restaurants weren't washing their hands after using the bathroom.[1]

I know this stuff isn't pleasant dinnertime conversation, but hygiene is part of the Great Physician's prescription. I've been influenced a great deal by the writings of Dr. Seaton, who said that advanced hygiene techniques are the single most important factor in maintaining good health. "All the vitamins, minerals, herbs, special diets, and exercise machines pale in comparison to hygiene. The Spartans in ancient Greece exercised to perfection, practiced the best possible diet, had no pollution and little stress, yet life expectancy was around twenty-six years of age," he wrote in his newsletter, *Hygiene & Health*. "Yet their society perished because of its failure to adopt good personal hygiene techniques."

What do those techniques look like?

I'm glad you asked because practicing advanced hygiene has become an everyday habit for me. Since I'm aware that 90 percent of germs take up residence around my fingernails, I use a creamy semisoft soap rich in essential oils. Each morning and evening, I dip both hands into the tub of semisoft soap and dig my fingernails into the cream. Then I work the special cream around the tips of fingers, cuticles, and fingernails for fifteen to thirty seconds. When I'm finished, I lather my hands for fifteen seconds before rinsing them under running water. After my hands are clean, I take another dab of semisoft soap and wash my face.

My second step involves a procedure that I call a facial dip. I fill my washbasin or a clean, large bowl with warm but not hot water. When enough water is in the basin, I add one-to-two tablespoons of regular table salt and two eyedroppers of a mineral-based facial solution into the cloudy water. I mix everything up with my hands, and then I bend over and dip my face into the cleansing matter, opening my eyes several times to allow the membranes to be cleansed. After coming up for air, I dunk my head a second time and blow bubbles through my nose. "Sink snorkeling," I call it.

My final two steps of advanced hygiene involve applying very diluted drops of hydrogen peroxide and minerals into my ears for thirty to sixty seconds to cleanse the ear canal, followed by brushing my teeth with an essential oil–based tooth solution to cleanse my teeth, gums, and mouth of unhealthy germs. (For more information on my favorite advanced hygiene products, visit www.BiblicalHealthInstitute.com and click on the GPRx Resource Guide.)

Following this advanced hygiene protocol involves discipline; you have to remind yourself to do it until it becomes an ingrained habit. I find it easier to follow these steps in the morning when I'm freshly awake rather than later in the evening

when I'm tired and bleary eyed—although I do my best to practice advanced hygiene morning and evening and hardly ever
miss. Either way, I know it takes only three minutes or so to
complete all of the advanced hygiene steps.

I urge you to incorporate advanced hygiene into your life,
paying attention to washing your hands periodically, especially
after you've been in public situations and shaken the hands of a
few friends. I don't want to drive up anyone's paranoia meter,
but sometimes our biggest exposure to germs all week happens
after church, when we're shaking hands with old friends and
new acquaintances in the foyer. All the while, we're exchanging
a garden variety of bacteria, allergens, environmental toxins, and
viruses from one part of the body to another.

Now, I know some people say they don't mind getting sick
because they lose a few pounds that way, but that's no way to get
a trim physique.

℞ THE GREAT PHYSICIAN'S Rx FOR WEIGHT LOSS: PRACTICE ADVANCED HYGIENE

- *Dig your fingers into a semisoft soap with essential
  oils and wash your hands regularly, paying special
  attention to removing germs from underneath your
  fingernails.*

- *Cleanse your nasal passageways and the mucous
  membranes of the eyes daily by performing a facial dip.*

- *Cleanse the ear canals at least twice per week.*

- *Use an essential oil-based tooth solution daily to remove germs from the teeth, gums, and mouth.*

Take Action

To learn how to incorporate the principles of practicing advanced hygiene, please turn to page 74 for the Great Physician's Rx for Weight Loss Battle Plan.

KEY #4

Condition Your Body
with Exercise and Body Therapies

Not that long ago people didn't have to plan to exercise. Life was synonymous with physical exertion, and we woke up in the morning with a full day of substantial bodily effort in front of us: performing back-breaking labor around the farm, tramping for miles to shop for daily provisions, or constantly moving around the factory floor. Male or female, we were on our feet all day, burning calories by the bushel.

These days, fewer and fewer lives are defined by physical activity. Planes, trains, and automobiles take us where we want to go in air-conditioned and seated comfort. Labor-saving inventions—from Cuisinarts to washing machines to moving walkways—make life easier, although I really think we use the extra time to cram more things into the day. What's happening is that we are in the midst of a historic shift from a manufacturing economy to a more service-oriented one. The information age has created sedentary jobs that require little, if any, physical effort.

To compound the problem of inactivity, our commutes involve more sitting (in a car), and once we're home, many of us retreat to the living room, where we're transformed into couch potatoes. Television viewing has been linked to excess weight in adults, including a study showing that women who watched three to four hours of TV per day were twice as likely to be overweight than those who watched less than one hour a day.[1]

To break a sweat today involves a conscious effort for us. Unless you're a UPS delivery person, you'll probably have to be intentional about exercising, even if that means scheduling an appointment with yourself to do so. Trying to lose weight without exercising would be like trying to ace a final exam without studying. While it can be done, ninety-nine times out of a hundred you can't lose weight—or at least sustain any weight loss—without stoking the body's furnace to burn up reserves of fat.

Let me do the math for you. If you're a male weighing 250 pounds, it's a physiological fact that to maintain your current weight, you must eat approximately twelve calories for every pound you weigh. (It's ten calories per pound for women.) For 250-pound males, this would mean eating 3,000 calories a day to maintain their weight. For a 170-pound woman, she would maintain her weight by eating 1,700 calories a day.

When you begin eating healthy, you stop consuming as many calories as before. You're eating foods created by God in a form healthy for the body, which contain fewer calories per bite than, for instance, a Big Mac value meal, which weighs in with 1,200 calories on the take-out tray. When you add exercise to your day, you *accelerate* your weight loss.

Working out in the gym each morning burns between 500 and 1,000 calories a day. If you work out faithfully five times a week, you should burn 3,500 calories. Since each pound of human fat is the equivalent of 3,500 calories, you can see that you'll lose at least one pound a week even if you maintain the same caloric intake. When you exercise faithfully *and* eat the right foods, however, you'll deliver a one-two punch against your heavyset ways.

If you haven't darkened the door of a neighborhood fitness center in ages, or the last time you exercised was running after a foul ball at your son's Little League game, then I know a great way to get back into the exercise game. It's called *functional fitness*, and this form of gentle exercise will get your body burning calories and improve agility. The idea behind functional fitness is to train movements, not muscles, as you build up cardiovascular endurance and the body's core muscles. You do this through performing real-life activities in real-life positions. For more information on functional fitness and to see detail descriptions of functional fitness exercises, visit www.GreatPhysiciansRx.com.

Functional fitness employs your own body weight as resistance, but you can also utilize dumbbells, mini trampolines, and stability balls. Classes in functional fitness are gaining popularity around the country. Instructors at LA Fitness, Bally Total Fitness, and local YMCAs put you through a series of exercises that mimic everyday life. You're asked to perform squats with feet apart, feet together, and one back with the other forward. You're asked to do reaching lunges, push-ups against a wall, and "supermans" that involve lying on the floor and lifting up your right arm while lifting your left leg into a fully extended position. You're *not* asked to perform high-impact exercises like those found in energetic, pulsating aerobics classes.

A functional fitness program provides an entry-level approach to exercise, increases strength in the daily tasks of life and, when done once or twice a day for five to fifteen minutes at a time, burns calories so that you can lose unwanted weight.

OTHER STRATEGIES

Here are some other body therapies to add to your arsenal.

Walk Up a Storm

Another fantastic form of exercise is walking, which is especially good for those who've been overweight for years and fear they're physically incapable of working out. This low-impact route to fitness is a surprisingly effective regimen for losing weight. Walking places a gentle strain on the hips and the rest of the body, and when done briskly, it makes the heart work harder and expend more energy.

Best of all, you can walk when it fits your schedule—before work, on your lunch hour, before dinner, or after dinner. You set the pace; you decide how much you put into this exercise. Walking is a social exercise that allows you to carry on a civilized conversation with a friend or loved one. There isn't anything better than my after-dinner walks with my wife, Nicki, as we push Joshua along in his stroller or I carry him in my backpack.

Go to Bed Earlier

Sleep is a body therapy in short supply these days. A nationwide "sleep deficit" means that we're packing in as much as we can from the moment we wake up until we crawl into bed sixteen, seventeen, or eighteen exhausting hours later. American adults are down to a little less than seven hours of sleep each night, a good two hours less than our great-great-grandparents slept a hundred years ago.

If you're looking to control your weight, sleep can help out. University of Chicago researchers found a link between the lack of sleep and the risk of weight gain. They were able to identify how a lack of sleep boosts the appetite, especially for high-calorie, high-carbohydrate foods. Sleep is a major regulator of leptin, a hormone that tells the brain that it doesn't need more food, and ghrelin, a different hormone that triggers hunger. When test subjects slept only four hours nightly, leptin levels decreased by 18 percent and ghrelin levels increased 28 percent.[2] Translation: they had the munchies for a midnight snack.

How many hours of sleep are you getting nightly? The magic number is eight hours, say the sleep experts. That's because when people are allowed to sleep as much as they would like in a controlled setting (such as a sleep laboratory), they naturally sleep eight hours in a twenty-four-hour time period.

Rest on the Seventh Day

In addition to proper sleep, the body needs a time of rest every seven days—a time to reboot, so to speak. This is accomplished by taking a break from the rat race on Saturday or Sunday. God created the earth and the heavens in six days and rested on the seventh, giving us an example and a reminder that we need to take a break from our labors. Just as triathletes and other superb athletes are careful to give their bodies one day off a week, we should be as well. Otherwise, we're prime candidates for burnout.

Let the Sun Shine In

You may not see much correlation between sunning yourself and losing weight, but let me explain. When your face or your arms and legs are exposed to sunlight, the skin synthesizes vitamin D from the ultraviolet rays of sunlight. The body needs vitamin D to produce adequate blood levels of insulin. When not enough insulin is present in the bloodstream, the body naturally wants to raise insulin levels, meaning that the brain sends out signals that it needs high-carbohydrate foods. Another factor is that exposure to sunlight can help your metabolism through normalization of thyroid function.

I recommend intentionally exposing yourself to at least fifteen minutes of sunlight a day to increase vitamin D levels in the body. That is often not possible because we're indoors during the day, or it's winter and the sun refuses to break through the gray cloud cover. That's why I recommend taking an omega-3 cod-liver oil complex, an important source of vitamin D. Cod-liver oil also helps prevent bone deterioration in adults, improves cardiovascular function, and contributes to long life. A teaspoon or three capsules a day are all you need.

Treat Yourself to Hydrotherapy

Hydrotherapy comes in the form of baths, showers, washing, and wraps—using hot *and* cold water. For instance, I wake up with a hot shower in the mornings, but then I turn off the hot water and stand under the brisk cold water for about a minute, which totally invigorates me. Cold water stimulates the body and boosts oxygen use in the cells, while hot water dilates blood vessels, which improves blood circulation and transports more oxygen to the brain.

You may be wondering if you can lose weight sitting in a sauna, which is a form of hydrotherapy. Yes, a sauna will cause you to shed a little weight, but that's water loss from perspiration, which means you'll gain weight right back as soon you replace those lost fluids. A session in the sauna will rid your body of toxins, however, and that's a good thing for any weight-loss regimen.

As a form of therapy, I also recommend a cold shower after taking a sauna, or—if you are really adventurous—running outside into a fresh blanket of snow. I did that once after sitting in a Vail hot tub until my skin was a bright pink. Then I ran outside into a freezing Rocky Mountain evening and rolled in the snow. Now that was invigorating!

The next time you shower, warm up your body first with hot water. Then slowly turn off the hot water until the cool water becomes cold. Stay under the cold nozzle for at least a minute. You'll feel an increase in energy while improving body awareness.

Pamper Yourself with Aromatherapy and Music Therapy

The final two body therapies elevate mood, which is certainly an issue when you're trying to lose weight. In aromatherapy, essential oils from plants, flowers, and spices can be introduced to your skin and pores either by rubbing them in or inhaling their aromas. The use of these essential oils will not miraculously shed pounds, but they will give you an emotional lift if you're struggling with hunger or other withdrawal-like pains. Try rubbing a few drops of myrtle, coriander, hyssop, galbanum, or frankincense onto the palms, then cup your hands over your mouth and nose and inhale. A deep breath will invigorate the spirit.

So will listening to soft and soothing music that promotes relaxation and healing. I know what I like when it comes to music therapy: contemporary praise and worship music. No matter what works for you, you'll find that listening to uplifting "mood" music can heal the body, soul, and spirit.

℞ THE GREAT PHYSICIAN'S Rx FOR WEIGHT LOSS: CONDITION YOUR BODY WITH EXERCISE AND BODY THERAPIES

- *Make a commitment and an appointment to exercise three times a week or more.*

- *Incorporate five-to-fifteen minutes of functional fitness into your daily schedule.*

- *Take a brisk walk and see how much better you feel at the end of the day.*

- *Make a conscious effort to practice deep-breathing exercises once a day. Inflate your lungs to full and hold for several seconds before slowly exhaling.*

- *Go to sleep earlier, paying close attention to how much sleep you get before midnight. Do your best to get eight hours of sleep nightly. Remember that sleep is the most important nonnutrient you can incorporate into your health regimen.*

- *End your next shower by changing the water temperature to cool (or cold) and standing underneath the spray for one minute.*

- *Next Saturday or Sunday, take a day of rest. Dedicate the day to the Lord and do something fun and relaxing that you haven't done in a while. Make your rest day work-free, errand-free, and shop-free. Trust God that He'll do more with His six days than you can do with seven.*

- *During your next break from work, sit outside in a chair and face the sun. Soak up the rays for ten or fifteen minutes.*

- *Incorporate essential oils into your daily life.*

- *Play worship music in your home, in your car, or on your iPod. Focus on God's plan for your life.*

Take Action

To learn how to incorporate the principles of conditioning your body with exercise and body therapies, please turn to page 74 for the Great Physician's Rx for Weight Loss Battle Plan.

Key #5

Reduce Toxins in Your Environment

I've been fortunate never to have gone on a diet.

Now, before you grab the nearest brick and toss it in my direction, hear me out. President Clinton once famously said, "I feel your pain," and I can declare that because I've put my body through three-day fasts. I know what it's like to experience light-headedness, dizzy spells, and an inability to concentrate on anything more than my next meal.

If you've struggled with your weight, then you've surely tried a few diets and experienced the same sense of deprivation. It doesn't matter what diet you've tried, be it Atkins to cabbage soup to grapefruit halves: by midafternoon you wish someone would stuff you into a wooden barrel and push you over Niagara Falls.

Physiologically there's a reason you feel horrible. The more fat cells that take up residence in your torso, the more toxins you've stored in your body. When you lose fat cells, you release toxins into your bloodstream, which are reabsorbed into the body. That's why you feel atrocious and search for the nearest couch to lie down on. Your emotional balance has been disrupted by toxins that have crossed the blood/brain barrier.

We have toxins inside our bodies because they are present everywhere in our environment—the air we breathe, the water we drink, the lotions and cosmetics we rub on our skin, the products we use to clean our home, and even the toothpaste we dab on our toothbrushes. If your blood and urine were tested, lab technicians would uncover dozens of toxins in your bloodstream, including PCBs (polychlorinated biphenyls), dioxins, furans, trace metals, phthalates, VOCs (volatile organic compounds), and chlorine.

Some toxins are water-soluble, meaning they are rapidly passed out of the body and present no harm. Unfortunately, many more toxins are fat-soluble, meaning that it can take months or years before they are completely eliminated from your system. Some of the more well-known fat-soluble toxins are dioxins, phthalates, and chlorine, and when they are not eliminated from the body, they become stored in your fatty tissues. "Consider those love handles as a hiding place for stored toxins and poisons," says Don Colbert, M.D. and author of *Toxic Relief.* "In other words, fat is usually toxic, too."[1]

The best way to flush fat-soluble toxins out of your bloodstream is to increase your intake of drinking water, which helps eliminate toxins through the kidneys (which I'll get into shortly). You must increase the fiber in your diet to eliminate toxins through the bowel, exercise and sweat to eliminate toxins through the lymphatic system, and practice deep breathing to eliminate toxins through the lungs.

Another way to reduce the number of toxins is to consume organic or grass-fed meat and dairy to reduce the number of toxins you take in. Remember: most commercially produced beef, chicken, and pork act as chemical magnets for toxins in the environment, so they will not be as healthy as eating grass-fed beef. In addition, consuming organic produce purchased at health food stores, roadside stands, and farmers' markets (only if produce is grown locally and unsprayed) will expose you to less pesticide residues, as compared to conventionally grown fruits and vegetables.

Canned tuna is another food to eat minimally, although many popular diets include tuna and salad as a lunchtime or dinner staple. Metallic particles of mercury, lead, and aluminum continue to be found in the fatty tissues of tuna, swordfish, and king mackerel. Shrimp and lobster, which are shellfish that scavenge the ocean floor, are unclean meats that should be eliminated from your diet. I recommend you limit the consumption of canned tuna to two cans per week and avoid shellfish completely.

WHAT TO DRINK

I've already touted the healthy benefits of drinking water, but when it comes to reducing toxins in your environment, water is especially important because of its ability to flush out toxins and other metabolic wastes from the body, and overweight people tend to have larger metabolic loads.

Increasing your intake of water will speed up your metabolism—which can lead to weight loss—and allow your body to assimilate nutrients from the foods you eat and the nutritional supplements you take. Since water is the primary resource for carrying nutrients throughout the body, a lack of adequate hydration results in metabolic wastes assaulting your body—a form of self-poisoning. That's why the importance of drinking enough water cannot be overstated: water is a life force involved in nearly every bodily process, from digestion to blood circulation.

Yet many eschew water for a pale imitation—soft drinks or diet drinks. According to a *U.S. News & World Report* feature, soft-drink consumption has quadrupled since 1950, from 11 gallons per year to about 46 gallons in 2003.[2] Let me do some computations: a gallon of Coke is 128 ounces, or around 10 12-ounce cans of Coke, to use a popular example. At 11 gallons per year in 1950, we were drinking 110 cans of Coke a year per capita, or about 1 Coke every three days. These days, we drink 46 gallons of Coke, or 460 cans, per year. That's more than 1 Coke per day—and 69,000 calories per year. Holy moly!

Regular sodas are sweetened with high fructose corn syrup because it's cheaper than using sucrose from sugar cane and beets, but high fructose corn syrup is more readily converted to fat, which is easily stored in the gut when excess calories are consumed. This is why *The Great Physician's Rx for Weight Loss* places a total ban on soft drinks.

The answer is not switching to diet soft drinks either, and beverages such as coffee, tea, and fruit juice do not count toward your water intake, even though they can be healthy for you. Diet drinks contain artificial sweeteners like aspartame, acesulfame K, or sucralose. Although the Food and Drug Administration has approved the use of artificial sweeteners in drinks (and food), these chemical food additives may prove to be detrimental to your health in the long term. And if you're thinking that energy drinks like Red Bull and Sobe Adrenaline Rush are a solution to hydration, then let me remind you that these drinks come "fortified" with caffeine and unhealthy additives.

Nothing beats plain old water—a liquid created by God to be

totally compatible with your body—especially when you're trying to lose weight. You should be drinking one quart of water for every fifty pounds of body weight, so if you weigh 250 pounds, you should be drinking more than one gallon of water daily.

I know what you're thinking: *Jordan, if I drink that much water, I can never be farther than fifteen steps from a bathroom.* Yes, you will probably treble your trips to the toilet, but trust me on this: if you're serious about losing weight, you must be serious about drinking enough water. There's no other physiological way for you to rid yourself of fat reserves and toxins stored inside your body.

Here's another reason why you should drink so much water: when the body is properly hydrated, the kidneys function normally, and the liver can convert stored fat into usable energy. In other words, the liver—acting like a traffic cop—will direct the body to tap into its fat reserves when (1) you're eating leaner, healthier foods and consuming less calories; and (2) you're exercising more.

You can greatly accelerate the liver's ability to convert stored fat into usable energy by consuming an abundance of clean, healthy water. Cold or lukewarm, it doesn't matter. Water helps you digest your meals more efficiently, reduces fluid retention, and prevents constipation. You'll also notice a difference in your skin as water reduces the appearance of wrinkles and gives the skin a healthy glow.

I don't recommend drinking water straight from the tap, however. Nearly all municipal water is routinely treated with chlorine or chloramine, potent bacteria-killing chemicals. I've installed a whole-house filtration system that removes the chlorine and other impurities from the water *before* it enters our household pipes. My wife, Nicki, and I can confidently turn on the tap and enjoy the health benefits of chlorine-free water for drinking, cooking, and bathing. Since our water doesn't have a chemical aftertaste, we're more apt to drink it.

If money is an issue, then consider installing inexpensive water filters at your kitchen sink or purchasing a countertop water pitcher with a built in carbon-based filter for less than twenty dollars. Installing a water filter means you'll be more apt to drink the water your body needs.

Toxins Elsewhere in Your Environment

Other toxins not directly related to weight loss are important enough to mention.

Plastics

Although I drink mineral waters from plastic containers when I'm not at home, I think it's safer to drink water from glass because of the presence of dioxins and phthalates added in the manufacturing process of plastic.

Air Quality

We spend 90 percent of our time indoors, usually in well-insulated and energy-efficient homes and offices with central air-conditioning in the summer and forced-air heating during the winter. Double-pane windows, when tamped down shut, don't allow any fresh air into the home and trap "used" air filled with harmful particles such as carbon dioxide, nitrogen dioxide, and pet dander.

Perhaps you've noticed all the attention given to mold-related illnesses and how homes have been torn up to rid walls and studs of spores of green and black mold. Those living in mold-infested environments have been diagnosed with impaired thyroid and adrenal problems, chronic fatigue, and memory impairment. It's tough to stick with a lifestyle change—or remember to do so—if poor indoor air quality drains your energy.

I recommend opening your doors and windows periodically to freshen the air you breathe, even if the temperatures are blazing hot or downright freezing. Just a few minutes of fresh air will do wonders.

I also recommend the purchase of a quality air filter, which will remove and neutralize tiny airborne particles of dust, soot, pollen, mold, and dander. I have set up four high-quality air purifiers in our home that scrub harmful impurities from the air.

Household Cleaners

Many of today's commercial household cleaners contain potentially harmful chemicals and solvents that expose people to VOCs (volatile organic compounds), which can cause eye, nose, and throat irritation.

Nicki and I have found that natural ingredients like vinegar, lemon juice, and baking soda are excellent substances that make our home spick-and-span. Natural cleaning products that aren't harsh, abrasive, or potentially dangerous to your family are available in grocery and natural food stores.

Skin Care and Body Care Products

Toxic chemicals such as chemical solvents and phthalates are found in lipstick, lip gloss, lip conditioner, hair coloring, hair spray, shampoo, and soap. Ladies, when you rub a tube of lipstick across your lips, your skin readily absorbs these toxins, and that's unhealthy. As with the case regarding household cleaners, you can find natural cosmetics in progressive natural food markets, although they are becoming more widely available in drugstores and beauty stores.

Let me add a word about toothpaste. A tube of toothpaste contains a warning that in case of accidental swallowing, you should contact the local Poison Control Center. What's that all about? Most commercially available toothpastes contain artificial sweeteners, potassium nitrate, and a whole bunch of long, unpronounceable words. Again, search out a healthy, natural version.

R̽ THE GREAT PHYSICIAN'S Rx FOR WEIGHT LOSS: REDUCE TOXINS IN YOUR ENVIRONMENT

- *Drink the recommended eight glasses of water daily—or one quart for every fifty pounds of body weight.*

- *Use glass containers instead of plastic containers whenever possible.*

- *Improve indoor air quality by opening windows and buying an air filtration system.*

- *Use natural cleaning products for your home.*

- *Use natural products for skin care, body care, hair care, cosmetics, and toothpaste.*

Take Action

To learn how to incorporate the principles of reducing toxins in your environment, please turn to page 74 for the Great Physician's Rx for Weight Loss Battle Plan.

KEY #6

Avoid Deadly Emotions

The stress of divorcing a wandering husband, owning her own insurance agency, and raising two preteen children came crashing all around Gidget Stous during the Christmas season of 2003. She reacted to the anxiety by snacking on Christmas cookies left in the lunchroom, eating every scrap of delicious food on her plate when she lunched with the "girls," and not denying herself at the holiday buffet tables. When Gidget finally gathered up the courage to look in a mirror, the sight of a twenty-seven-year-old woman who had let herself go too far horrified her.

She reluctantly stepped on the scale and gasped at her weight: 230 pounds. What a mess her life had become! Her doctor pronounced her a borderline diabetic—type 2—and diagnosed her with a case of adult ADHD, prompting him to prescribe a pair of strong meds—Paxil and Adderall. She quickly became addicted to both drugs, which acted as stimulants.

Her chart revealed other afflictions: acid reflux, allergies, hypertension, elevated cholesterol levels, and a "female problem"—endometriosis. "I had really low energy, was miserable, and terribly stressed about everything happening in my life," she told me after I met her while speaking at a church in Kansas City, Missouri.

Things began to turn around when she began dating a fellow named Michael. Her boyfriend gave her one of my earlier books to read—*The Maker's Diet,* but she put the book aside for several months until she finally began reading it one evening.

When she came to the section on how I don't eat pork because God didn't design our bodies to eat scavenger animals, Gidget's immediate reaction was, "No way." She had an emotional attachment to bacon on her breakfast plate and pork chops with mashed potatoes and gravy for dinner. That was how she was raised.

But as she took stock, she remembered what her doctor had said during her last visit: "Gidget, you have the cholesterol level of a sixty-five-year-old woman. If you don't do something soon, you won't see your children grow up."

After she married Michael, she took the Bible's health advice to heart and realized immediate results. The advanced hygiene program of morning and evening facial dips took care of her allergies. She exchanged the half-dozen Cokes she drank at her desk for bottled water. She stopped eating processed foods and unclean meats. She and Michael and the children even volunteered to do chores at a nearby farm in exchange for raw milk, free-range eggs, real butter, and grass-fed beef and chicken.

In less than six months, she lost eighty-five pounds. "Many of my longtime customers at the office didn't recognize me when I got down to 140 pounds. After the extra weight went away, so did my stress," Gidget told me.

There was another deadly emotion, however, that Gidget had to deal with, and it was unforgiveness. This is common for those who grew up tubby or flabby. Perhaps you were teased unmercifully in the schoolyard, called names like "Lard Butt" or

"Fatso." When you reached adulthood, the digs were delivered in a more subtle form: "Are you really going to eat that?" or "Have you thought about trying this diet?"

"Adults were the most insensitive to me," Gidget said. "They'd make these little remarks while they were eating the same junk in the lunchroom."

Gidget did something that I recommend for those dealing with unforgiveness in their hearts. She wrote down the names of those who had hurt her and each grievance they had brought against her. Then she asked God to help her forgive them, followed by crumpling up the paper and tossing it into the trash. "I had issues with people who were mean to me, including family members," Gidget said. "One way or another, I had to forgive them because otherwise I'd become too stressed over the whole thing."

What about you? Are you harboring resentment in your heart, nursing a grudge into overtime, or plotting revenge against those who hurt you? If you're still bottling up emotions such as anger, bitterness, and resentment, these deadly emotions will produce toxins similar to bingeing on a dozen glazed doughnuts. The efficiency of your immune system decreases noticeably for six hours, and staying angry and bitter about those who have teased you in the past can alter the chemistry of your body—and even prompt you to fall off the healthy food wagon again. An old proverb states it well: "What you are eating is not nearly as important as what's eating you."

This is not the time to revert to old habits: consuming a deep-dish large pizza in one sitting, scarfing a package of Oreo cookies, or plying yourself with "pleasure" foods filled with fat and sugar, such as a box of Mrs. See's candy or a Baskin-Robbins banana split. If you're still annoyed by those who teased you about your body shape, made snide comments about your plus-size clothes, or told you that you'll never lose weight, you have to let it go. Sure, they were mean to you, but that's history.

As much as she had been hurt, Gidget put her past in the rearview mirror and moved forward. Following the Great Physician's Rx for a healthy lifestyle helped her deal with the deadly emotions weighing her down. As for you, please remember that no matter how badly you've been hurt in the past, it's still possible to forgive. "If you forgive men their trespasses, your heavenly Father will also forgive you," Jesus said. "But if you do not forgive men their trespasses, neither will your Father forgive your trespasses" (Matt. 6:14–15).

Give your forgiveness to those who tormented you, hurt you, and made you angry, and then let it go.

R℞ THE GREAT PHYSICIAN'S Rx FOR WEIGHT LOSS: AVOID DEADLY EMOTIONS

- *Don't eat when you're sad, scared, or angry.*

- *Recognize the interaction between deadly emotions and being overweight.*

- *Trust God when you face circumstances that cause you to worry or become anxious.*

- *Practice forgiveness every day and forgive those who hurt you.*

Take Action

To learn how to incorporate the principles of avoiding deadly emotions, please turn to page 74 for the Great Physician's Rx for Weight Loss Battle Plan.

KEY #7

Live a Life of Prayer and Purpose

Alan Jones had a nightly routine that he *loved:* plopping down on the couch after the boys were put to bed and scarfing heaping scoops of his favorite ice cream. In three nights Alan could polish off a half-gallon. Each ice-cream-palooza was chased with a cup of coffee.

In his youthful days, Alan could eat those gooey desserts without adding a pound to his athletic frame, but after passing forty a few years ago, his torso thickened as a slower middle-age metabolism kicked in. His weight gain happened so slowly that he barely noticed the additional thirty pounds. Whereas his ideal weight had been around 165 pounds, now he was pushing 195. Even at this weight Alan didn't look grossly overweight; he merely resembled the typical American male who was just a little . . . out of shape.

Two things transpired during a one-month time span that turned around Alan's life. The first marker cropped up when he submitted to his annual physical. While his blood pressure had always been a rock-solid 120/80, this time his doctor tsked-tsked when he announced the latest results: 140/90.

The second event occurred when Alan heard me speak at my home church, Christ Fellowship in Palm Beach Gardens, where Alan is the media pastor in charge of sound, lights, and production. That evening, I asked—well, you can say I strongly

urged—the pastors and the staff of Christ Fellowship to participate in a forty-day trial study following the Great Physician's
Rx for weight loss.

Alan raised his hand and agreed to give it a shot. He was gen-
erally concerned about his lack of energy, high blood pressure,
and low desire to exercise. I asked those participating in the trial
study to write an entrance essay and an exit essay describing
their thoughts. Here's an excerpt from Alan's entrance essay:

> My wife, Cinda, says I can start a project better than
> anyone else she knows—it's the finishing part that
> doesn't win any blue ribbons. After careful considera-
> tion, I realized that she was right, especially when it
> came to losing weight. I always have great anticipation
> for the wonderful results, but I have seldom had the
> discipline to stick with it. This time will be different. My
> goal is to bring my body to the proper balance and to
> correct my higher blood pressure. I have two young
> boys, Matthew and Henry, watching whether their dad
> will faithfully see this to the end. I'll be praying that this
> time I'll really turn things around.

I like what Alan had to say about prayer because it should be
foundational to every Christian endeavor. This time, Alan stuck
with the program. I'll let him describe the changes that forty
days brought:

Wow, I'm amazed by the changes in my body after following the Great Physician's Rx for weight loss. My blood pressure is back to its normal 120/80 status, and I've lost twenty pounds, which has prompted people to plead with me to share my "secret." I've heard comments like, "You look ten years younger," and "You're the incredible shrinking man."

Now I'm so aware of the foods I eat. Fast-food restaurants really have no appeal to me. God changed my desire for my nightly ice cream ritual, and I have discovered the joy of the treadmill and Rollerblading. I mentioned in my Entrance essay how important it was for me to finish this not only for myself, but for my two little men. They are proud of their daddy and have been so encouraging. Thank you, Jordan, for helping me understand that one of my purposes in life is being around for Matthew and Henry, ages fourteen and ten.

What I enjoy most about his story is that Alan *got* it. He understood that the key to unlocking his health potential was based on having a purpose—getting healthy so that he'll be around for his wife and kids. Since writing his Exit essay, he's lost another ten pounds and is down to 165.

When and if you decide to adopt the principles found in *The Great Physician's Rx for Weight Loss* for your life, I urge you to undergird your effort with prayer as Alan did, which will give you the perseverance to complete what you start. Seal all that you do with the power of prayer, and watch your life become more than you ever thought possible.

> ### Start a Small Group
>
> It's difficult to face the battle of the bulge alone. If you have friends or family members struggling with excess pounds, ask them to join you in following the Great Physician's Rx for weight loss. To learn about joining an existing group in the area or leading a small group in your church, please visit www.GreatPhysiciansRx.com.

I'm not guaranteeing that miraculous things will happen to you or your loved ones, although they often do. But I will tell you that if you treat your body as God meant for you to treat it—like a temple of the Holy Spirit (1 Cor. 6:19–20)—God will honor that.

You know, people ask me if overeating is a sin. While the Bible has little direct criticism of gluttony, the book of Proverbs describes the social and economic disadvantages of gluttony, which is defined as excess in eating and drinking. "Do not mix with winebibbers, or with gluttonous eaters of meat; for the drunkard and the glutton will come to poverty, and drowsiness will clothe a man with rags," says Proverbs 23:20-21.

Here's where I come down on the topic. If you're wondering

whether you can overeat and still get to heaven, my response is yes, you'll get to heaven. You'll just get there a lot sooner.

When you follow God's health plan, however, you'll honor your family, and the best way to honor them is by staying here on earth. I always cringe when I hear about someone involved in ministry—the pastorate, the mission field, or even lay ministry—who dies way too early because he did not take care of his body. That's a waste of God's most precious resource here on earth, His children.

God has a purpose for your life, and when you're called to serve Him in ministry, every minute is precious. Every year we have more to offer, not less, because we have wisdom and experience on our side. Use that wisdom by establishing a health legacy for your future generations, and you won't live a life of regrets.

You may be reading this and thinking, *I don't look as good as I used to . . . I can tell when people are staring at me.* Well, you've been given the knowledge to do something about your health and excess weight from this day forward. How are you going to act upon what you've learned from *The Great Physician's Rx for Weight Loss?*

It matters, you know. I lost both my grandfathers way too early: My grandfather on my father's side was significantly overweight and died at the age of sixty-two from a heart attack. My grandfather on my mother's side was overweight as well, and he died of a heart attack at the age of fifty-five. Both of my grandfathers were gone before I turned ten years old.

You don't have to die early. Give yourself the best chance to be there for your loved ones by following the seven keys found in *The Great Physician's Rx for Weight Loss.*

℞ THE GREAT PHYSICIAN'S Rx FOR WEIGHT LOSS: LIVE A LIFE OF PRAYER AND PURPOSE

- *Pray continually.*

- *Confess God's promises upon waking and before you retire.*

- *Find God's purpose for your life and live it.*

- *Be an agent of change in your life. Only you can take that first step toward weight loss.*

Take Action

To learn how to incorporate the principles of living a life of prayer and purpose, please turn to page 74 for the Great Physician's Rx for Weight Loss Battle Plan.

THE GREAT PHYSICIAN'S RX
FOR WEIGHT LOSS BATTLE PLAN

Upon Waking

Prayer: thank God because this is the day that the Lord has made. Rejoice and be glad in it. Thank Him for the breath in your lungs and the life in your body. Ask the Lord to heal your body and use your experience to benefit the lives of others. Read Matthew 6:9–13 out loud.

Purpose: ask the Lord to give you an opportunity to add significance to someone's life today. Watch for that opportunity. Ask God to use you this day for His intended purpose.

Advanced hygiene: for hands and nails, jab fingers into semisoft soap four or five times, and lather hands with soap for fifteen seconds, rubbing soap over cuticles and rinsing under water as warm as you can stand it. Take another swab of semisoft soap into your hands and wash your face. Next, fill basin or sink with water as warm as you can stand it, and add one-to-three tablespoons of table salt and one-to-three eyedroppers of iodine-based mineral solution. Dunk face into water and open eyes, blinking repeatedly underwater. Keep eyes open underwater for three seconds. After cleaning your eyes, put your face back in the water, and close your mouth while blowing bubbles out of your nose. Come up from the water, and immerse your face in the water once again, gently taking water into your nostrils and expelling bubbles. Come up from the water, and blow your nose into facial tissue. To cleanse the ears, use hydrogen peroxide and mineral-based ear drops, putting two or three drops into each ear and letting stand for sixty seconds. Tilt your head to expel the drops. For the teeth, apply two or three drops of essential oil-based tooth drops to the toothbrush. This can be used to brush your teeth or added to existing toothpaste. After brushing your teeth, brush your tongue for fifteen seconds. (For recommended advanced hygiene products, visit www.BiblicalHealthInstitute.com and click on the GPRx Resource Guide.)

Reduce toxins: open your windows for one hour today. Use natural soap and natural skin and body care products (shower gel, body creams, etc.). Use natural facial care products. Use natural toothpaste. Use natural hair care products such as shampoo, conditioner, gel, mousse, and hairspray (for recommended products, visit www.BiblicalHealthInstitute.com and click on the GPRx Resource Guide).

Supplements: take one serving of a fiber/green superfood powder (mixed) or five caplets of a super green formula swallowed with twelve-to-sixteen ounces of water (for recommended products, visit www.BiblicalHealthInstitute.com and click on the GPRx Resource Guide).

Body therapy: get twenty minutes of direct sunlight sometime during the day, but be careful between the hours of 10:00 a.m. and 2:00 p.m.

Exercise: perform functional fitness exercises for five to fifteen minutes or spend five to fifteen minutes on a mini trampoline. Finish with five to ten minutes of deep-breathing exercises. (One to three rounds of the exercises can be found at www.GreatPhysiciansRx.com.)

Emotional health: whenever you face a circumstance, such as your health, that causes you to worry, repeat the following: "Lord, I trust You. I cast my cares upon You, and I believe that You're going to take care of [insert your current situation] and make my health and make my body strong." Confess that throughout the day whenever you think about the condition of your health.

Breakfast

Make a smoothie in a blender with the following ingredients: one cup plain yogurt or kefir (goat's milk is best); one tablespoon organic flaxseed oil; one tablespoon organic raw honey; one cup of organic fruit (berries, banana, peaches, pineapple, etc.); two tablespoons goat's milk protein powder (visit www.BiblicalHealthInstitute.com and click on the GPRx Resource Guide for recommendations); dash of vanilla extract (optional)

Supplements: take two whole food multivitamin caplets and one capsule of a whole food antioxidant/energy formula (see the GPRx Resource Guide on page TK for recommended products).

Lunch

Before eating, drink eight ounces of water.

During lunch, drink eight ounces of water or hot tea (for recommended products, visit www.BiblicalHealthInstitute.com and click on the GPRx Resource Guide) with honey.

large green salad with mixed greens, avocado, carrots, cucumbers, celery, tomatoes, red cabbage, red peppers, red onions, and sprouts with three hard-boiled omega-3 eggs

salad dressing: use extra virgin olive oil, apple cider vinegar or lemon juice, Celtic sea salt, herbs, and spices, or mix one tablespoon of extra virgin olive oil with one tablespoon of a healthy store-bought dressing

one apple with skin

Supplements: take two whole food multivitamin caplets and one capsule of a whole food antioxidant/energy formula.

Dinner

Before eating, drink eight ounces of water.

During dinner, drink hot tea with honey.

baked, poached, or grilled wild-caught salmon

steamed broccoli

large green salad with mixed greens, avocado, carrots, cucumbers, celery, tomatoes, red cabbage, red onions, red peppers, and sprouts

salad dressing: use extra virgin olive oil, apple cider vinegar or lemon juice, Celtic sea salt, herbs, and spices, or mix one tablespoon of extra virgin olive oil with one tablespoon of a healthy store-bought dressing

Supplements: take two whole food multivitamin caplets and one capsule of a whole food antioxidant blend and one-to-three teaspoons or three-to-nine capsules of a high omega-3 cod-liver oil complex (for recommended products, visit www.BiblicalHealthInstitute.com and click on the GPRx Resource Guide).

Snacks

apple slices with raw sesame butter (tahini)

one whole food nutrition bar with beta-glucans from soluble oat fiber (for recommended products, visit www.BiblicalHealthInstitute.com and click on the GPRx Resource Guide)

Drink eight-to-twelve ounces of water, or hot or iced fresh-brewed tea with honey.

Before Bed

Exercise: go for a walk outdoors or participate in a favorite sport or recreational activity.

Supplements: take one serving of a fiber/green superfood powder (mixed) or five caplets of a super green formula swallowed with twelve-to-sixteen ounces of water.

Body therapy: take a warm bath for fifteen minutes with eight drops of biblical essential oils added (for recommended products, visit www.BiblicalHealthInstitute.com and click on the GPRx Resource Guide).

Advanced hygiene: repeat the advanced hygiene instructions from the morning of Day 1.

Emotional health: ask the Lord to bring to your mind someone you need to forgive. Take out a sheet of paper and write the person's name at the top. Try to remember each specific action that person did against you that brought you pain. Write down the following: "I forgive [insert person's name] for [insert the action he or she did against you]." After you fill up the paper, tear it up or burn it, and ask God to give you the strength to truly forgive that person.

Purpose: ask yourself these questions: *Did I live a life of purpose today? What did I do to add value to someone else's life today?* Commit to living a day of purpose tomorrow.

Prayer: thank God for this day, asking Him to give you a restoring night's rest and a fresh start tomorrow. Thank Him for His steadfast love that never ceases and His mercies new every morning. Read Romans 8:35, 37–39 out loud.

Sleep: go to bed by 10:30 p.m.

Day 2

Upon Waking

Prayer: thank God because this is the day that the Lord has made. Rejoice and be glad in it. Thank Him for the breath in your lungs and the life in your body. Ask the Lord to heal your body and use your experience to benefit the lives of others. Read Psalm 91 out loud.

Purpose: ask the Lord to give you an opportunity to add significance to someone's life today. Watch for that opportunity. Ask God to use you this day for His intended purpose.

Advanced hygiene: follow the advanced hygiene recommendations from the morning of Day 1.

Reduce toxins: follow the recommendations to reduce toxins from the morning of Day 1.

Supplements: take one serving of a fiber/green superfood powder (mixed) or five caplets of a super green formula swallowed with twelve-to-sixteen ounces of water.

Body therapy: take a hot and cold shower. After a normal shower, alternate sixty seconds of water as hot as you can stand it, followed by sixty seconds of water as cold as you can stand it. Repeat the cycle four times for a total of eight minutes, finishing with cold.

Exercise: perform functional fitness exercises for five to fifteen minutes or spend five to fifteen minutes on a mini trampoline. Finish with five to ten minutes of deep-breathing exercises. (One to three rounds of the exercises can be found at www.GreatPhysiciansRx.com.)

Emotional health: follow the emotional health recommendations from the morning of Day 1.

Breakfast

two or three eggs any style, cooked in one tablespoon of extra virgin coconut oil

stir-fried onions, mushrooms, and peppers

one slice of sprouted or yeast-free whole grain bread with almond butter and honey

Supplements: take two whole food multivitamin caplets and one capsule of a whole food antioxidant/energy formula.

Lunch

Before eating, drink eight ounces of water.

During lunch, drink eight ounces of water or hot tea with honey.

large green salad with mixed greens, avocado, carrots, tomatoes, red cabbage, red onions, red peppers, and sprouts with three ounces of cold, poached, or canned wild salmon salad dressing: use extra virgin olive oil, apple cider vinegar or lemon juice, Celtic sea salt, herbs, and spices, or mix one tablespoon of extra virgin olive oil with one tablespoon of a healthy store-bought dressing

organic grapes

Supplements: take two whole food multivitamin caplets and one capsule of a whole food antioxidant/energy formula.

Dinner

Before eating, drink eight ounces of water.

During dinner, drink hot tea with honey.

roasted organic chicken

cooked vegetable (carrots, onions, peas, etc.)

large green salad with mixed greens, avocado, carrots, tomatoes, red cabbage, red onions, red peppers, and sprouts

salad dressing: use extra virgin olive oil, apple cider vinegar or lemon juice, Celtic sea salt, herbs, and spices, or mix one tablespoon of extra virgin olive oil with one tablespoon of a healthy store-bought dressing

Supplements: take two whole food multivitamin caplets and one capsule of a whole food antioxidant/energy blend and one-to-three teaspoons or three-to-nine capsules of a high omega-3 cod-liver oil complex.

Snacks

raw almonds and apple wedges

one whole food nutrition bar with beta-glucans from soluble oat fiber

Drink eight-to-twelve ounces of water, or hot or iced fresh-brewed tea with honey.

Before Bed
Exercise: go for a walk outdoors or participate in a favorite sport or recreational activity.

Supplements: take one serving of a fiber/green superfood powder (mixed) or five caplets of a super green formula swallowed with twelve-to-sixteen ounces of water.

Advanced hygiene: repeat the advanced hygiene instructions from the morning of Day 1.

Emotional health: repeat the emotional health recommendations from the evening of Day 1.

Purpose: ask yourself these questions: *Did I live a life of purpose today? What did I do to add value to someone else's life today?* Commit to living a day of purpose tomorrow.

Prayer: thank God for this day, asking Him to give you a restoring night's rest and a fresh start tomorrow. Thank Him for His steadfast love that never ceases and His mercies that are new every morning. Read 1 Corinthians 13:4–8 out loud.

Body therapy: spend ten minutes listening to soothing music before you retire.

Sleep: go to bed by 10:30 p.m.

DAY 3

Upon Waking
Prayer: thank God because this is the day that the Lord has made. Rejoice and be glad in it. Thank Him for the breath in your lungs and the life in your body. Ask the Lord to heal your body and use your experience to benefit the lives of others. Read Ephesians 6:13–18 out loud.

Purpose: ask the Lord to give you an opportunity to add significance to someone's life today. Watch for that opportunity. Ask God to use you this day for His intended purpose.

Advanced hygiene: follow the advanced hygiene recommendations from the morning of Day 1.

Reduce toxins: follow the recommendations to reduce toxins from the morning of Day 1.

Supplements: take one serving of a fiber/green superfood powder (mixed) or five caplets of a super green formula swallowed with twelve-to-sixteen ounces of water.

Body therapy: get twenty minutes of direct sunlight sometime during the day, but be careful between the hours of 10:00 a.m. and 2:00 p.m.

Exercise: perform functional fitness exercises for five to fifteen minutes or spend five to fifteen minutes on a mini trampoline. Finish with five to ten minutes of deep-breathing exercises. (One to three rounds of the exercises can be found at www.GreatPhysiciansRx.com.)

Emotional health: follow the emotional health recommendations from the morning of Day 1.

Breakfast

four-to-eight ounces of organic whole milk yogurt or cottage cheese with fruit (pineapple, peaches, or berries), honey, and a dash of vanilla extract

handful of raw almonds

one cup of hot tea with honey

Supplements: take two whole food multivitamin caplets and one capsule of a whole food antioxidant/energy formula.

Lunch

Before eating, drink eight ounces of water.

During lunch, drink eight ounces of water or hot tea with honey.

large green salad with mixed greens, avocado, carrots, cucumbers, celery, tomatoes, red cabbage, red peppers, red onions, and sprouts with two ounces of low mercury, high omega-3 canned tuna (for recommended products, visit www.BiblicalHealthInstitute.com and click on the GPRx Resource Guide.)

salad dressing: use extra virgin olive oil, apple cider vinegar or lemon juice, Celtic sea salt, herbs, and spices, or mix one tablespoon of extra virgin olive oil with one tablespoon of a healthy store-bought dressing

one piece of fruit in season

Supplements: take two whole food multivitamin caplets and one capsule of a whole food antioxidant/energy formula.

Dinner

Before eating, drink eight ounces of water.

During dinner, drink hot tea with honey.

red meat steak (beef, buffalo, or venison)

steamed broccoli

baked sweet potato with butter

large green salad with mixed greens, avocado, carrots, cucumbers, celery, tomatoes, red cabbage, red peppers, red onions, and sprouts

salad dressing: use extra virgin olive oil, apple cider vinegar or lemon juice, Celtic sea salt, herbs, and spices, or mix one tablespoon of extra virgin olive oil with one tablespoon of a healthy store-bought dressing

Supplements: take two whole food multivitamin caplets and one capsule of a whole food antioxidant/energy blend and one-to-three teaspoons or three-to-nine capsules of a high omega-3 cod-liver oil complex.

Snacks

four ounces of whole milk yogurt with fruit, honey, and a few almonds one whole food nutrition bar with beta-glucans from soluble oat fiber

Drink eight-to-twelve ounces of water, or hot or iced fresh-brewed tea with honey.

Before Bed

Exercise: go for a walk outdoors or participate in a favorite sport or recreational activity.

Supplements: take one serving of a fiber/green superfood powder (mixed) or five caplets of a super green formula swallowed with twelve-to-sixteen ounces of water.

Body therapy: take a warm bath for fifteen minutes with eight drops of biblical essential oils added.

Advanced hygiene: follow the advanced hygiene instructions from the morning of Day 1.

Emotional health: follow the forgiveness recommendations from the evening of Day 1.

Purpose: ask yourself these questions: *Did I live a life of purpose today? What did I do to add value to someone else's life today?* Commit to living a day of purpose tomorrow.

Prayer: thank God for this day, asking Him to give you a restoring night's rest and a fresh start tomorrow. Thank Him for His steadfast love that never ceases and His mercies that are new every morning. Read Philippians 4:4–8, 11–13, 19 out loud.

Sleep: go to bed by 10:30 p.m.

DAY 4

Upon Waking

Prayer: thank God because this is the day that the Lord has made. Rejoice and be glad in it. Thank Him for the breath in your lungs and the life in your body. Read Matthew 6:9–13 out loud.

Purpose: ask the Lord to give you an opportunity to add significance to someone's life today. Watch for that opportunity. Ask God to use you this day for His intended purpose.

Advanced hygiene: follow the advanced hygiene recommendations from the morning of Day 1.

Reduce toxins: follow the recommendations for reducing toxins from the morning of Day 1.

Supplements: take one serving of a fiber/green superfood powder (mixed) or five caplets of a super green formula swallowed with twelve-to-sixteen ounces of water.

Exercise: perform functional fitness exercises for five to fifteen minutes or spend five to fifteen minutes on a mini trampoline. Finish with five to ten minutes of deep-breathing exercises. (One to three rounds of the exercises can be found at www.GreatPhysiciansRx.com.)

Body therapy: take a hot and cold shower. After a normal shower, alternate sixty seconds of water as hot as you can stand it, followed by sixty seconds of water as cold as you can stand it. Repeat cycle four times for a total of eight minutes, finishing with cold.

Emotional health: follow the emotional health recommendations from the morning of Day 1.

Breakfast
three soft-boiled or poached eggs

four ounces of sprouted whole grain cereal with two ounces of whole milk yogurt or goat's milk (for recommended products, visit www.BiblicalHealthInstitute.com and click on the GPRx Resource Guide)

one cup of hot tea with honey

Supplements: take two whole food multivitamin caplets and one capsule of a whole food antioxidant/energy formula.

Lunch

Before eating, drink eight ounces of water.

During lunch, drink eight ounces of water or hot tea with honey.

large green salad with mixed greens, avocado, carrots, cucumbers, celery, tomatoes, red cabbage, red peppers, red onions, and sprouts with two ounces of low mercury, high omega-3 canned tuna

salad dressing: use extra virgin olive oil, apple cider vinegar or lemon juice, Celtic sea salt, herbs, and spices, or mix one tablespoon of extra virgin olive oil with one tablespoon of a healthy store-bought dressing

one bunch of grapes with seeds

Supplements: take two whole food multivitamin caplets and one capsule of a whole food antioxidant/energy formula.

Dinner

Before eating, drink eight ounces of water.

During dinner, drink hot tea with honey.

grilled chicken breast

steamed veggies

small portion of cooked whole grain (quinoa, amaranth, millet, or brown rice) cooked with one tablespoon of extra virgin coconut oil

large green salad with mixed greens, avocado, carrots, cucumbers, celery, tomatoes, red cabbage, red peppers, red onions, and sprouts

salad dressing: use extra virgin olive oil, apple cider vinegar or lemon juice, Celtic sea salt, herbs, and spices, or mix one tablespoon of extra virgin olive oil with one tablespoon of a healthy store-bought dressing.

Supplements: take two whole food multivitamin caplets and two capsules of a whole food antioxidant blend and one-to-three teaspoons or three-to-nine capsules of a high omega-3 cod-liver oil complex.

Snacks

apple and carrots with raw almond butter

one whole food nutrition bar with beta-glucans from soluble oat fiber

Drink eight-to-twelve ounces of water, or hot or iced fresh-brewed tea with honey.

Before Bed

Drink eight-to-twelve ounces of water or hot tea with honey.

Exercise: go for a walk outdoors or participate in a favorite sport or recreational activity.

Supplements: take one serving of a fiber/green superfood powder (mixed) or five caplets of a super green formula swallowed with twelve-to-sixteen ounces of water.

Advanced hygiene: follow the advanced hygiene recommendations from the morning of Day 1.

Emotional health: follow the forgiveness recommendations from the evening of Day 1.

Purpose: ask yourself these questions: *Did I live a life of purpose today? What did I do to add value to someone else's life today?* Commit to living a day of purpose tomorrow.

Prayer: thank God for this day, asking Him to give you a restoring night's rest and a fresh start tomorrow. Thank Him for His steadfast love that never ceases and His mercies that are new every morning. Read Romans 8:35, 37–39 out loud.

Body therapy: spend ten minutes listening to soothing music before you retire.

Sleep: go to bed by 10:30 p.m.

DAY 5 (PARTIAL-FAST DAY)

Upon Waking

Prayer: thank God because this is the day that the Lord has made. Rejoice and be glad in it. Thank Him for the breath in your lungs and the life in your body. Read Isaiah 58:6–9 out loud.

Purpose: ask the Lord to give you an opportunity to add significance to someone's life today. Watch for that opportunity. Ask God to use you this day for His intended purpose.

Advanced hygiene: follow the advanced hygiene recommendations from the morning of Day 1.

Reduce toxins: follow the recommendations for reducing toxins from the morning of Day 1.

Supplements: take one serving of a fiber/green superfood powder (mixed) or five caplets of a super green formula swallowed with twelve-to-sixteen ounces of water.

Exercise: perform functional fitness exercises for five to fifteen minutes or spend five to fifteen minutes on a mini trampoline. Finish with five to ten minutes of deep-breathing exercises. (One to three rounds of the exercises can be found at www.GreatPhysiciansRx.com.)

Body therapy: get twenty minutes of direct sunlight sometime during the day, but be careful between the hours of 10:00 a.m. and 2:00 p.m.

Emotional health: follow the emotional health recommendations from the morning of Day 1.

Breakfast

none (partial-fast day)

Drink eight-to-twelve ounces of water.

Supplements: take two whole food multivitamin caplets and one capsule of a whole food antioxidant/energy formula.

Lunch

Drink eight-to-twelve ounces of water.

none (partial-fast day)

Supplements: take two whole food multivitamin caplets and one capsule of a whole food antioxidant/energy formula.

Dinner

Before eating, drink eight ounces of water.

During dinner, drink hot tea with honey.

Chicken Soup

cultured vegetables (for recommended products, visit www.BiblicalHealthInstitute.com and click on the GPRx Resource Guide)

large green salad with mixed greens, avocado, carrots, cucumbers, celery, tomatoes, red cabbage, red peppers, red onions, and sprouts

salad dressing: use extra virgin olive oil, apple cider vinegar or lemon juice, Celtic sea salt, herbs, and spices, or mix one tablespoon of extra virgin olive oil with one tablespoon of a healthy store-bought dressing

Supplements: take two whole food multivitamin caplets and two capsules of a whole food antioxidant blend and one-to-three teaspoons or three-to-nine capsules of a high omega-3 cod-liver oil complex.

Snacks

none (partial-fast day)

Drink eight ounces of water.

Before Bed

Drink eight-to-twelve ounces of water or hot tea with honey.

Exercise: go for a walk outdoors or participate in a favorite sport or recreational activity.

Supplements: take one serving of a fiber/green superfood powder (mixed) or five caplets of a super green formula swallowed with twelve-to-sixteen ounces of water.

Advanced hygiene: follow the advanced hygiene recommendations from the morning of Day 1.

Emotional health: follow the forgiveness recommendations from the evening of Day 1.

Body therapy: take a warm bath for fifteen minutes with eight drops of biblical essential oils added.

Purpose: ask yourself these questions: *Did I live a life of purpose today? What did I do to add value to someone else's life today?* Commit to living a day of purpose tomorrow.

Prayer: thank God for this day, asking Him to give you a restoring night's rest and a fresh start tomorrow. Thank Him for His steadfast love that never ceases and His mercies that are new every morning. Read Isaiah 58:6–9 out loud.

Sleep: go to bed by 10:30 p.m.

DAY 6 (REST DAY)

Upon Waking

Prayer: thank God because this is the day that the Lord has made. Rejoice and be glad in it. Thank Him for the breath in your lungs and the life in your body. Read Psalm 23 out loud.

Purpose: ask the Lord to give you an opportunity to add significance to someone's life today. Watch for that opportunity. Ask God to use you this day for His intended purpose.

Advanced hygiene: follow the advanced hygiene recommendations from the morning of Day 1.

Reduce toxins: follow the recommendations for reducing toxins from the morning of Day 1.

Supplements: take one serving of a fiber/green superfood powder (mixed) or five caplets of a super green formula swallowed with twelve-to-sixteen ounces of water.

Exercise: no formal exercise since it's a rest day.

Body therapies: none since it's a rest day.

Emotional health: follow the emotional health recommendations from the morning of Day 1.

Breakfast

two or three eggs cooked any style in one tablespoon of extra virgin coconut oil

one grapefruit or orange

handful of almonds

Supplements: take two whole food multivitamin caplets and one capsule of a whole food antioxidant/energy formula.

Lunch

Before eating, drink eight ounces of water.

During lunch, drink eight ounces of water or hot tea with honey.

large green salad with mixed greens, avocado, carrots, cucumbers, celery, tomatoes, red cabbage, red peppers, red onions, and sprouts with three hard-boiled omega-3 eggs

salad dressing: use extra virgin olive oil, apple cider vinegar or lemon juice, Celtic sea salt, herbs, and spices, or mix one tablespoon of extra virgin olive oil with one tablespoon of a healthy store-bought dressing

one organic apple with the skin

Supplements: take two whole food multivitamin caplets and one capsule of a whole food antioxidant/energy formula.

Dinner

Before eating, drink eight ounces of water.

During dinner, drink hot tea with honey.

roasted organic chicken

cooked vegetables (carrots, onions, peas, etc.)

large green salad with mixed greens, carrots, cucumbers, celery, tomatoes, red cabbage, red peppers, red onions, and sprouts

salad dressing: use extra virgin olive oil, apple cider vinegar or lemon juice, Celtic sea salt, herbs, and spices, or mix one tablespoon of extra virgin olive oil with one tablespoon of a healthy store-bought dressing.

Supplements: take two whole food multivitamin caplets and two capsules of a whole food antioxidant/energy blend and one-to-three teaspoons or three-to-nine capsules of a high omega-3 cod-liver oil complex.

Snacks

handful of raw almonds with apple wedges

one whole food nutrition bar with beta-glucans from soluble oat fiber

Drink eight-to-twelve ounces of water, or hot or iced fresh-brewed tea with honey.

Before Bed

Drink eight-to-twelve ounces of water or hot tea with honey.

Exercise: go for a walk outdoors or participate in a favorite sport or recreational activity.

Supplements: take one serving of a fiber/green superfood powder (mixed) or five caplets of a super green formula swallowed with twelve-to-sixteen ounces of high-alkaline water or raw vegetable juice.

Advanced hygiene: follow the advanced hygiene recommendations from the morning of Day 1.

Emotional health: follow the forgiveness recommendations from the evening of Day 1.

Purpose: ask yourself these questions: *Did I live a life of purpose today? What did I do to add value to someone else's life today?* Commit to living a day of purpose tomorrow.

Prayer: thank God for this day, asking Him to give you a restoring night's rest and a fresh start tomorrow. Thank Him for His steadfast love that never ceases and His mercies that are new every morning. Read Psalm 23 out loud.

Body therapy: spend ten minutes listening to soothing music before you retire.

Sleep: go to bed by 10:30 p.m.

DAY 7

Upon Waking

Prayer: thank God because this is the day that the Lord has made. Rejoice and be glad in it. Thank Him for the breath in your lungs and the life in your body. Read Psalm 91 out loud.

Purpose: ask the Lord to give you an opportunity to add significance to someone's life today. Watch for that opportunity. Ask God to use you this day for His intended purpose.

Advanced hygiene: follow the advanced hygiene recommendations from the morning of Day 1.

Reduce toxins: follow the recommendations for reducing toxins from the morning of Day 1.

Supplements: take one serving of a fiber/green superfood powder (mixed) or five caplets of a super green formula swallowed with twelve-to-sixteen ounces of water.

Exercise: perform functional fitness exercises for five to fifteen minutes or spend five to fifteen minutes on a mini trampoline. Finish with five to ten minutes of deep-breathing exercises. (One to three rounds of the exercises can be found at www.GreatPhysiciansRx.com.)

Body therapy: get twenty minutes of direct sunlight sometime during the day, but be careful between the hours of 10:00 a.m. and 2:00 p.m.

Emotional health: follow the emotional health recommendations from the morning of Day 1.

Breakfast

Make a smoothie in a blender with the following ingredients: one cup plain yogurt or kefir (goat's milk is best); one tablespoon organic flaxseed oil; one tablespoon organic raw honey; one cup of organic fruit (berries, banana, peaches, pineapple, etc.); two tablespoons goat's milk protein powder; dash of vanilla extract (optional)

Supplements: take two whole food multivitamin caplets and one capsule of a whole food antioxidant/energy formula.

Lunch

Before eating, drink eight ounces of water.

During lunch, drink eight ounces of water or hot tea with honey.

large green salad with mixed greens, raw goat cheese, avocado, carrots, cucumbers, celery, tomatoes, red cabbage, red peppers, red onions, and sprouts with three ounces of cold, poached, or canned wild-caught salmon

salad dressing: use extra virgin olive oil, apple cider vinegar or lemon juice, Celtic sea salt, herbs, and spices, or mix one tablespoon of extra virgin olive oil with one tablespoon of a healthy store-bought dressing one piece of fruit in season

Supplements: take two whole food multivitamin caplets and one capsule of a whole food antioxidant/energy formula.

Dinner

Before eating, drink eight ounces of water.

During dinner, drink hot tea with honey.

baked or grilled fish of your choice

steamed broccoli

baked sweet potato with butter

large green salad with mixed greens, carrots, cucumbers, celery, tomatoes, red cabbage, red peppers, red onions, and sprouts

salad dressing: use extra virgin olive oil, apple cider vinegar or lemon juice, Celtic sea salt, herbs, and spices, or mix one tablespoon of extra virgin olive oil with one tablespoon of a healthy store-bought dressing

Supplements: take two whole food multivitamin caplets and one capsule of a whole food antioxidant/energy blend and one-to-three teaspoons or three-to-nine capsules of a high omega-3 cod-liver oil complex.

Snacks

apple slices with raw sesame butter (tahini)

one whole food nutrition bar with beta-glucans from soluble oat fiber

Drink eight-to-twelve ounces of water, or hot or iced fresh-brewed tea with honey.

Before Bed

Drink eight-to-twelve ounces of water or hot tea with honey.

Exercise: go for a walk outdoors or participate in a favorite sport or recreational activity.

Supplements: take one serving of a fiber/green superfood powder (mixed) or five caplets of a super green formula swallowed with twelve-to-sixteen ounces of high-alkaline water or raw vegetable juice.

Advanced hygiene: follow the advanced hygiene recommendations from the morning of Day 1.

Emotional health: follow the forgiveness recommendations from the evening of Day 1.

Body therapy: take a warm bath for fifteen minutes with eight drops of biblical essential oils added.

Purpose: ask yourself these questions: *Did I live a life of purpose today? What did I do to add value to someone else's life today?* Commit to living a day of purpose tomorrow.

Prayer: thank God for this day, asking Him to give you a restoring night's rest and a fresh start tomorrow. Thank Him for His steadfast love that never ceases and His mercies that are new every morning. Read 1 Corinthians 13:4–8 out loud.

Sleep: go to bed by 10:30 p.m.

DAY 8 AND BEYOND

If you're beginning to lose weight and feel better, but still have more pounds to lose on your road to wellness, you can repeat the Great Physician's Rx for Weight Loss Battle Plan as many times as you'd like. For detailed step-by-step suggestions and meal and lifestyle plans, visit www.GreatPhysiciansRx.com and join the 40- Day Health Experience if you want to continue to lose weight rapidly. Or you may be interested in the Lifetime of Wellness plan if you want to maintain your newfound level of health. These online programs will provide you with customized daily meal and exercise plans and provide you the tools to track your progress.

If you've experienced positive results from the Great Physician's Rx for Weight Loss program, I encourage you to reach out to people you know and recommend this book and program to them. You can learn how to lead a small group at your church or home by visiting www.GreatPhysiciansRx.com.

Remember: you don't have to be a doctor or a health expert to help transform the life of someone you care about—you just have to be willing.

Allow me to offer this prayer of blessing from Numbers 6:24–26 for you:

> May the Lord bless you and keep you.
> May the Lord make His face to shine upon you and be
>   gracious unto you.
> May the Lord lift up His countenance upon you and bring
>   you peace.
> In the name of Yeshua Ha Mashiach, Jesus our Messiah.
> Amen.

Need Recipes?

For a detailed list of more than two hundred healthy and delicious recipes contained in the Great Physician's Rx eating plan, please visit www.GreatPhysiciansRx.com.

NOTES

Introduction

1. S.J. Olshansky, D.J. Passaro, and R.C. Hershow, et al., "A Potential Decline in Life Expectancy in the United States in the 21st Century," *New England Journal of Medicine*, 352:11, 1138–1145.

2. Keep in mind that physicians commit themselves, on average, to six to eight years of arduous medical school study and resident training before they enter public or private practice, but during all those years of classroom study and hands-on training, these would-be physicians take just *one* nine-week class in nutrition. Check the following Web sites: http://www.catalogs.umn.edu/tcmed/curric.html and http://som.georgetown.edu/curriculum/Curr_chart_2003-04-1.pdf.

3. Lindsey Tanner, "Obesity Surgery Riskier Than Once Thought, New Research Finds," Associated Press, October 19, 2005.

4. Gus Prosch Jr., M.D., "The Truth and Fallacies About Obesity," *Alternative Medicine: The Definitive Guide,* ed. Larry Trivieri Jr. (Berkeley, CA: Celestial Arts, 2002), 822.

5. *Encyclopedia of Natural Healing* (Burnaby, B.C.: Alive Publishing Group, 1997), 1017.

Key #1

1. Rex Russell, M.D., *What the Bible Says About Healthy Living* (Ventura, CA: Regal, 1996), 63.

2. From the Mayo Clinic Web site, http://www.mayoclinic.com/health/diabetes-diet/DA00070.

3. *San Diego Union Tribune,* Sports section, May 12, 2005.

4. F. Batmanghelidj, M.D., *You're Not Sick, You're Thirsty!* (New York: Warner Books, 2003), 225–26.

5. "Slender Servings," *Experience Life,* May 2005, 20.

Key #3

1. "Foodborne Illness," published October 25, 2005, by the Centers for Disease Control and Prevention and the National Center for Infectious Diseases/Division of Bacterial and Mycotic Diseases and available online at http://www.cdc.gov/ncidod/dbmd/diseaseinfo/foodborneinfections_g.htm.

Key #4

1. In one study of 4,771 working women whose average age was thirty-five, Larry A. Tucker, Ph.D., professor and director of health promotion at Brigham Young University in Provo, Utah, discovered that those who spent more than three to four hours a day watching television had twice the risk of being obese as women who watched less than one hour daily.

2. Nanci Hellmich, "Sleep Loss May Equal Weight Gain," *USA Today,* December 6, 2004, http://www.usatoday.com/news/health/2004-12-06-sleep-weight-gain_x.htm.

Key #5

1. Don Colbert, *Toxic Relief* (Lake Mary, FL: Siloam, 2003), 15.

2. Elizabeth Querna, "One Sweet Nation," *U.S. News & World Report,* March 28, 2005, http://www.usnews.com/usnews/health/articles/050328/28sugar.b.htm.

ABOUT THE AUTHORS

Jordan Rubin has dedicated his life to transforming the health of others one life at a time. He is the founder and chairman of Garden of Life, Inc., a health and wellness company based in West Palm Beach, Florida, that produces whole food nutritional supplements and personal care products. He is also president and CEO of GPRx, Inc., a biblically based health and wellness company providing educational resources, small group curriculum, functional foods, nutritional supplements, and wellness services.

He and his wife, Nicki, married in 1999 and are the parents of a toddler-aged son, Joshua. They make their home in Palm Beach Gardens, Florida.

Joseph D. Brasco, M.D., who is board certified in internal medicine and gastroenterology, is in private practice in Indianapolis, Indiana. He has skillfully combined diet, supplementation, and judicious use of medications to provide a comprehensive and effective treatment program. Dr. Brasco is the coauthor of *Restoring Your Digestive Health* with Jordan Rubin.

The Great Physician's Rx DVD and Study Guide

LEARN AND APPLY 7 TIPS TO GOOD HEALTH

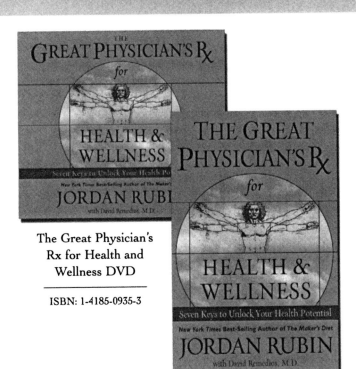

The Great Physician's
Rx for Health and
Wellness DVD

ISBN: 1-4185-0935-3

NELSON IMPACT
A Division of Thomas Nelson Publishers
Since 1798

www.thomasnelson.com

The Great Physician's
Rx for Health and
Wellness Study Guide

ISBN: 1-4185-0934-5

BHI

BIBLICAL HEALTH
INSTITUTE

The Biblical Health Institute (www.BiblicalHealthInstitute.com) is an online learning community housing educational resources and curricula reinforcing and expanding on Jordan Rubin's Biblical Health message.

Biblical Health Institute provides:

1. "101" level **FREE**, introductory courses corresponding to Jordan's book The Great Physician's Rx for Health and Wellness and its seven keys; Current "101" courses include:

   * "Eating to Live 101"

   * "Whole Food Nutrition Supplements 101"

   * "Advanced Hygiene 101"

   * "Exercise and Body Therapies 101"

   * "Reducing Toxins 101"

   * "Emotional Health 101"

   * "Prayer and Purpose 101"

2. **FREE** resources (healthy recipes, what to E.A.T., resource guide)

3. **FREE** media--videos and video clips of Jordan, music therapy samples, etc.--and much more!

Additionally, Biblical Health Institute also offers in-depth courses for those who want to go deeper.

Course offerings include:

   * 40-hour certificate program to become a Biblical Health Coach

   * A la carte course offerings designed for personal study and growth (launching late April 2006)

   * Home school courses developed by Christian educators, supporting home-schooled students and their parents (designed for middle school and high school ages—launching in August 2006).

For more information and updates on these and other resources go to
www.BiblicalHealthInstitute.com

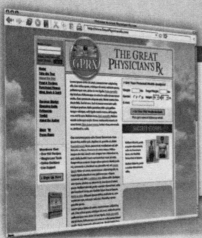

Lightning Source UK Ltd.
Milton Keynes UK
12 January 2010

148471UK00001B/23/P